Women and Borderline
Personality Disorder

Women
and Borderline
Personality Disorder

Symptoms and Stories

JANET WIRTH-CAUCHON

RUTGERS UNIVERSITY PRESS
New Brunswick, New Jersey, and London

Library of Congress Cataloging-in-Publication Data

Wirth-Cauchon, Janet, 1959–
    Women and borderline personality disorder: symptoms and stories /
Janet Wirth-Cauchon.
        p. cm.
    Includes bibliographical references and index.
    ISBN 0-8135-2890-9 (cloth: alk. paper) — ISBN 0-8135-2891-7 (pbk. :
alk. paper)
        1. Borderline personality disorder. 2. Women—Mental health—
Sociological aspects. 3. Women—Socialization. 4. Sex role—Psychological
aspects. I. Title.

RC569.5.B67 W57 2001
616.85'0082—dc21   00-039037

British Cataloging-in-Publication data for this book is available from the British
Library

An earlier version of chapter 2 appeared as "Colonizing the Borderland:
Deconstructing the Borderline in Psychiatry," in *Perspectives on Social Problems*,
vol. 11, edited by James A. Holstein and Gale Miller (Greenwich, Conn.: JAI
Press, 1997).

Selections from *Love's Executioner and Other Tales of Psychotherapy* by Irvin D.
Yalom, copyright © 1989 by Irvin D. Yalom, are reprinted by permission of Perseus
Books, L.L.C., New York.

Second paperback printing, 2003

Manufactured in the United States of America

To Judy

Contents

Acknowledgments

This project owes its existence to the energy and support of many people without whom it would not have come to life. First I must thank those at Boston College, where this project first took shape: I thank Stephen Pfohl, my dissertation chairperson, for his encouragement and invitation to dialogue, which has shaped my sociological identity and provoked the themes pursued in this book. The other members of my doctoral committee, Sharlene Hesse-Biber, Paul Breines, Jeanne Guilleman, and Eve Spangler, provided warm encouragement and thoughtful criticism during numerous conversations. I also benefited from the care and support of my dissertation study group, Janet Boguslaw, Mary-Ellen Boyle, and Elizabeth Sherman, and from the intellectual companionship and friendship of Emily Kearns, Tom Ryan, Larry Zaborski, Jackie Orr, Avery Gordon, Hope Lafferty, and Ann Murphy.

The transformation of this project from dissertation to book was a challenging one, and colleagues at Drake University, including Andrew Herman, Joseph Schneider, Vibeke Petersen, Min-Zhan Lu, and Bruce Horner, have provided guidance, encouragement, and new life to this project. They have also read portions of this manuscript and have given both substantive and editorial suggestions. My colleagues in the sociology, anthropology, and geography departments must be given special thanks for their support and for the creation of a uniquely collegial and supportive intellectual environment. I thank Marcie Gilliland for providing her expertise as well as materials that helped inform my analysis. I also thank the many students in my "Women, Madness, and Culture" and "Feminist Theory" courses, with whom I have explored the nuances of the themes of this project.

I must acknowledge the Center for the Humanities here at Drake University, which provided funding for the completion of this book. I also thank my acquiring editor at Rutgers, David Myers, for his continual encouragement and enthusiasm for this project.

Finally, I must acknowledge my family, including my parents, Stanley and Mary Cauchon, for their many years of love and support; and to Alex and Anne Marie, whose constant encouragement and love sustains my courage and animates this work: Thank you for your countless sacrifices both large and small that make this work possible, and that constitute love in its many forms.

Women and Borderline
Personality Disorder

Chapter 1

Women and the New Self Disorders

In *Borderline: Vision and Healing*, psychoanalyst Nathan Schwartz-Salant describes a woman patient whose condition he had diagnosed as borderline personality disorder:

> There is a strange, uncomfortable, somewhat inhuman feeling
> to her. It feels somewhat like having a dream with an archaic
> figure who speaks in a stilted language from a distant century,
> yet carries a strong affect. She speaks to me in plain English,
> has affects I clearly recognize, is suffering, yet also seems
> inhuman, of a different species. Her words carry a fullness that
> feels like they each link to greater whole, yet they are expressed
> in a strangely shallow manner. Alternatively, she has great
> depth and insight. But each moment is strained, too full and
> also too empty. She seems an outcast, living on the fringes of
> the world, cast into a dark shadow of inhuman, archetypal
> processes and speaking through them as if she were partaking of
> a human dialogue. She seems a princess, a witch, a clown, a
> trickster. We are in a fairy tale world of abstract characters
> which quickly turn back to flesh and blood reality. I am left
> feeling guilty for ever thinking of her as anything other than
> genuine. (1989, 9)

This analyst's troubled musings about his patient reveal the way psychoanalysts and psychotherapists imagine, struggle to understand, and tell stories about their experiences with patients deemed "border-line." The patient's status as not quite human, "of a different species"; the strained and strange affect that charges the room and Schwartz-Salant's relations to her; the fragmented and mutable characters that he imagines her to be: These images rhetorically place the woman deemed borderline in the shadows, on the "fringes of the world." Two major themes stand out: first, the patient's marginality to the human community, as patients are deemed to be located in a "no-man's-land" of ambiguity and chaos, a "borderland"; and second, the patient's frag-mented, continually changing, unstable self.

This book is a feminist interpretive analysis of the "borderline" cat-egory within psychoanalysis and psychiatry. It examines the interrelated issues of gender meanings, psychiatric knowledge, and women's experi-ence through a study of the social construction of this new "female malady" of late modern society, borderline personality disorder. The book is based on an interpretive study of case narratives and the psy-choanalytic frameworks that inform them, as well as of autobiographi-cal accounts by women diagnosed as borderline. I also trace the history of the meanings of the borderline concept in psychiatry and psycho-analysis. This analysis focuses on the language of selfhood in the dis-course on the borderline patient, examining how selves deemed unstable are represented as pathological, and how dominant gender ideologies of femininity shape this representation of women's madness.

As a story told by the interpreter, the psychoanalytic case study is, as critics of Freud's narratives of cases of hysteria point out, "a vivid record of the construction of [cultural assumptions] as they emerge from the desire of the interpreter" (Kahane 1985, 24–25). Stories of the treat-ment of personality disorders are sites where the negotiation of the meaning of selfhood, gender, and psychic disturbance is played out. As feminist critics of psychoanalysis have shown, psychoanalytic narratives have long been the sites where gender subjectivity—particularly that of women—is contested and produced. The case histories of hysterical women patients—Breuer and Freud's Anna O, Freud's Dora—are per-haps the paradigmatic instance of the cultural representation of female subjectivity through narrative (Cixous and Clément 1986; Gallop 1982; Irigaray 1985). The post-Freudian psychoanalytic and psychotherapeutic narratives of borderline personality disorders constitute a set of texts as yet largely unexamined from a feminist critical perspective.

The borderline construct, as its history shows, is a focal point for inconsistencies and contradictions within psychiatric knowledge. Because the borderline diagnosis is located literally at the borders between diagnostic categories, it is particularly reflective of central conflicts in psychiatric taxonomy, theory, and practice. As a category based on a metaphor of the border, it is "holographic," providing a condensed image of the larger culture of psychiatry. As D. Emily Hicks writes of the border metaphor in literature, "In the same way that one part of a hologram can produce an entire image, the border metaphor is able to reproduce the whole culture to which it refers" (Hicks 1991, xxix). The borderline is a site of contention, controversy, and struggle over boundaries, not only between the categories of disorder, but of the boundaries of madness itself, and of the limits of psychiatry.

The term "borderline" was first used in 1938 by analyst Adolph Stern to describe patients who appeared more severely disturbed than the neurotics that Freud felt were suitable for psychoanalysis, yet who did not show signs of outright psychosis, placing them, as Stern wrote, on "the border line between neurosis and psychosis" (Stern 1938, 467). These patients appeared to be more profoundly disturbed than those suffering neurotic symptoms, yet they could not be classified as psychotic. Stern felt that such patients showed signs of regressing to an early narcissistic state in which they had withdrawn libidinal energy from the outside world and turned it upon themselves. Hence, such patients showed evidence of pre-oedipal conflicts having to do with the earliest acquisition of a self, rather than the oedipal conflicts of neurotic patients.

Within contemporary psychiatric discourse, the borderline diagnosis acquired an official definition when it first appeared in the third edition of the Diagnostic and Statistical Manual of Mental Disorders, or DSM-III (APA 1980, revised in 1987), where it was defined as a personality disorder, characterized by "a pervasive pattern of instability of self-image, interpersonal relationships, and mood, beginning in early adulthood and present in a variety of contexts" (APA 1987, 346). A central feature of borderline personality disorder in the DSM definition is the appearance of an identity disturbance: "A marked and persistent

identity disturbance is almost invariably present. This is often pervasive, and is manifested by uncertainty about several life issues, such as
self-image, sexual orientation, long-term goals or career choice, types
of friends or lovers to have, or which values to adopt. The person often experiences this instability of self-image as chronic feelings of emptiness or boredom" (346).

By 1984, four years after its entry into the DSM in 1980, it had
become "by far the most common personality disorder," according to
researchers John Gunderson and Mary Zanarini, accounting for "15%
to 25% of hospital and outpatient cases" (Gunderson and Zanarini 1987,
8). In addition, the proportion of patients diagnosed with BPD who are
women has grown to an estimated 72 percent in the general population, and 70 to 77 percent in treatment settings (Becker 1997; Castaneda and Franco 1985; Gibson 1991; Gunderson and Zanarini 1987;
Swartz et al. 1990). Dana Becker argues that the borderline diagnosis
has been "feminized" and that borderline personality disorder has become a new "female malady" for the late twentieth century (Becker
1997, 24).

I first encountered the borderline diagnosis when I was a research
analyst with the Massachusetts Department of Mental Health. While
abstracting information from clinical records for a research project on
patients with exceptionally frequent admissions to one of the state psychiatric hospitals, I encountered several records with the diagnosis of
"borderline personality disorder." These stood out to me, not only
because these were the only case records in which the admitting diagnosis had been a personality disorder, but also because all of these borderline patients were young women who were described as having
identity confusions and turbulent past histories. One more item from
the records caught my attention: In almost every case, these young
women engaged in self-cutting—a form of self-injury that is common
for borderline patients.

The constellation of images—the preponderance of young women,
the identity disturbances, the self-cutting, and particularly the word
"borderline" itself, ambiguous and referential, piqued my curiosity. Who
were these young women? What caused their violent self-harm? And
what did "borderline" refer to—what border did these troubled young
women occupy?

This book is an outcome of my attempt to answer these questions. My inquiry has led in unexpected directions, however, as seemingly every attempt to determine the identity of the borderline patient has led to more than one answer, and to many more questions. The meaning of the term has proved elusive; it was different in each description I read. Eventually I realized that these changing meanings in psychiatric discourse are not necessarily distortions or obfuscations to its true meaning, but rather constitute the multiple and shifting "truths" of this term. As Michael Stone has written of the borderline concept, "Its history is its meaning" (Stone, in Cauwels 1992, 361).

And yet, within those shifting meanings, the growing predominance of women among those diagnosed as borderline is one prominent, though not often discussed, consistency. Prior to Dana Becker's recent comprehensive clinical study of women and borderline personality disorder (see also Linehan 1993), this gender specificity, with rare exceptions (Gibson 1991; Samuels 1988), was not directly discussed in the literature. Yet it proved to be a pattern in the case narratives of patients receiving the borderline diagnosis. This book explores the feminization of the borderline concept in psychoanalytic psychiatry. It focuses on the role of gender meanings in the psychoanalytic conceptualization of the borderline disorder and examines how the meaning of borderline disorder is rhetorically accomplished in psychiatric discourse and in case narratives of particular patients where the label "borderline" is deployed. My concern is with the recirculation within psychiatric texts of what Carol Cohn calls "gender discourse," which she defines as "a symbolic system, a central organizing discourse of culture, one that not only shapes how we experience and understand ourselves as men and women, but that also interweaves with other discourses and shapes them—and therefore shapes other aspects of our world" (Cohn 1995, 132).

Another prominent theme in the discourse on the borderline is the borderline patient's unstable, fragmented, or even missing self. In psychotherapeutic discourse, women deemed borderline are not only placed "on the borders," at the edges of sanity; they are also placed at the very margins of selfhood. Their selves are described as "dead" (Schwarz-Salant 1989), or "empty" (Singer 1977a), as "unstable" or "split" among "part-selves" (Flax 1986), as containing a "defect in the organizing structure of the self" (Ross 1976); alternatively, such patients are said to manifest a "blurring of ego boundaries" (that is, confusion between one's own thoughts and feelings and those of others) (Boyer 1977, 403).

This study is a cultural feminist analysis of the multiple meanings of the concept of an unstable, fragmented self, focusing on women's historic cultural identity and social positioning as a crucial context for a consideration of the significance of the borderline patient's crisis of selfhood. Here I draw upon feminist and sociological theories of subjectivity to examine the contradictions of feminine identity as it is represented and lived in late modern culture (Butler 1990; Butler 1993; de Lauretis 1984; Irigaray 1985).

Judith Butler writes of the relation between gender and self: "It would be wrong to think that the discussion of 'identity' ought to proceed prior to a discussion of gender identity for the simple reason that persons only become intelligible through becoming gendered in conformity with recognizable standards of gender intelligibility" (Butler 1990, 16).

Butler's critique of presocial conceptions of identity and subjecthood argues for the inseparability of gender and identity. They cannot be separated; to speak of "selves" necessarily draws one into a consideration of gender. Butler thus calls into question the neutrality and universality of the notion of "self." Her analysis is part of the feminist critique of the gendered quality of self, a dialogue that has challenged the "false universal" of the Western generic self. Feminist analyses have shown how conceptions of the self or subject are conflated with conceptions of masculine subjectivity, reflecting the experiences, desires, and illusions of this masculine position. At the same time, women have been constructed as Other, overdetermined by their feminine position in the gender binaries of patriarchal logic (Beauvoir 1989; Cixous and Clément 1986; Irigaray 1985).

Within this binary logic of self and other and of masculine and feminine, the status of feminine identity is unstable. Women's relation to the Western generic self has been marked by paradox and contradiction. Of crucial concern for this analysis is women's borderline status, in representational terms, between cultural conceptions of feminine identity and generic selfhood. Women are in a representational and experiential double bind—caught between two ideologies, that of a traditional essentialist feminine identity, on one hand, and the psychologically defined norm or ideal of healthy, normal selfhood, on the other. Ambiguity and confusion surround this double bind. What is femininity? What is its relation, as a construct, to dominant conceptions of "normal," generic selfhood? How has this relation changed under the impact of feminist recrafting of selfhood for women?

It is important to stress that this is not simply a theoretical problem of reconciling the conflicts between competing definitions of selfhood. As gender relations change and as masculinity and femininity become redefined, boundaries between the genders shift, creating areas of ambiguity. While these ambiguities are manifest in more formal epistemological and theoretical questions, they are also manifest in material relations between the sexes. They have an impact on people's everyday sense of themselves as gendered beings. The gender/self ambiguities are, in other words, experiential ambiguities. An exploration of the psychic breakdown in the self in borderline women, as well as of the ways this self breakdown is defined and interpreted by psychoanalysts and psychiatrists, reveals those cultural contradictions in particularly graphic form. Thus borderline symptoms and their interpretation become a text for the sociological study of gender, culture, and the self.

In her historical study of women and madness, Elaine Showalter has shown the deep symbolic association of madness with femininity in the history of Western society, which Showalter attributes to "a cultural tradition that represents 'woman' *as* madness and that uses images of the female body . . . to stand for irrationality in general" (Showalter 1985, 4). Feminist philosophers and social theorists have analyzed the gender dualism of this cultural tradition: "They have shown how women, within our dualistic systems of language and representation, are typically situated on the side of irrationality, silence, nature, and body, while men are situated on the side of reason, discourse, culture and mind" (Showalter 1985, 4).

Jane Ussher considers the entanglements of the meanings of gender and madness and points to the ways in which "the discourses which regulate femininity, 'woman' and 'the mad' are irrevocably linked" (Ussher 1992, 13). "Madness," she writes, "acts as a signifier which positions women as ill, as outside, as pathological, as somehow second-rate—the second sex. The scientific and cultural practices which produce the meanings and 'truths' about madness adopt the signifier 'madness' as the means of regulating and positioning women within the social order" (12).

The signifier par excellence in the past two centuries that positioned women as pathological and irrational, of course, was hysteria. Numerous feminist and historical analyses have documented the ways that discourses of hysteria were imbricated in gender ideologies of the nineteenth and early twentieth centuries (Bernheimer and Kahane 1985; Cixous and Clément 1986; Showalter 1985; Smith-Rosenberg 1972). The diagnosis of hysteria is an extreme, and by now obsolete, example of pathologization of women. Its broad inclusive aggregation of symptoms has been recategorized under other diagnoses (Herman 1992; Satow 1980).

However, there has been an increasing recognition among feminist observers that the label "borderline" may function in the same way that "hysteria" did in the late nineteenth and early twentieth century as a label for women. Mary Ann Jimenez, for example, writes, "The similarities between the diagnoses of borderline personality disorder and hysteria are striking. Both diagnoses delimit appropriate behavior for women, and many of the criteria are stereotypically feminine" (Jimenez 1997, 163). Dana Becker similarly compares borderline disorder with past conceptions of hysteria: "There is a malignant kinship between hysteria, as it was conceived of and treated during the latter part of the nineteenth century, and current conceptualizations and treatment of borderline personality disorder. This sisterhood is rooted in similarities in the way these two 'women's diseases' and the women who suffered from them are viewed" (Becker 1997, 19). Both diagnostic categories were defined as including an expanding number of symptoms over time, making their meaning heterogeneous and diffuse. Yet Jimenez points out that borderline is a more aggressive version of hysteria: "What distinguishes borderline personality disorder from hysteria is the inclusion of anger and other aggressive characteristics, such as shoplifting, reckless driving, and substance abuse. If the hysteric was a damaged woman, the borderline woman is a dangerous one" (Jimenez 1997, 163).

Noting the lack of attention to gender in the clinical literature on borderline personality disorder, Becker argues for analyses that address the "woman question" in relation to the borderline diagnosis. "How does the fact of the preponderance of women in this diagnostic category relate to the vagueness of the diagnostic criteria? How does it relate to the tailoring of the criteria to fit women? Why do more women than men display so-called borderline symptoms? Many books written about treatment of BPD do not, despite using women primarily as case examples, discuss gender in relation to the borderline diagnosis" (Becker 1997, xv).

Becker and Jimenez call on feminist scholars to take borderline personality disorder seriously as an important new category through which to view women's emotional distress.

The Empty Self: A New Type of Patient?

Women diagnosed as borderline present a crisis in subjective feelings about themselves. They may describe feeling empty, unreal, numb, or even nonexistent (Chessick 1972; Singer 1977a). One borderline patient's description of herself illustrates with particular force this sense of invisibility: "I'm afraid of being abandoned by other people, since I long ago abandoned myself. So there's no *one* there when I'm alone" (Yalom and Elkin 1974, 11).

The increase in the number of patients voicing complaints related to uncertainty about identity has led many analysts to mark a change in the types of patients they see, "from people concerned with troubling unconscious desires, as in the classical images [of Freudian analysis] . . . to people desperately seeking for a secure core of self" (Frosh 1991, 45).

Norman Lazar, for example, reported in 1973 that there had been a shift in the types of patients seeking analysis at the Columbia University Psychoanalytic Clinic, from the symptom neuroses to character disorders, particularly those involving problems in the sense of identity. Lazar asserted that "we no longer see the hysterics described in the early literature." Instead, there had been a "widening of the application of analysis to include increasingly severe degrees of character disorder, borderline cases, and some psychotics" (Lazar 1973, 584). Problems frequently mentioned by analysts included, according to Lazar, "impoverishment of affect and avoidance of commitment; permanent adolescence with fading of adulthood as an aim; omnipotent and narcissistic expectations . . . defective sense of identity; feelings of alien-ation and unrelatedness . . . and a compelling need for change, action, movement, immediacy, and 'fluidity'" (585–586).

Other analysts noted that patients more frequently expressed their problems as problems with their sense of self, suffering from what ana-lyst Melvin Singer described as a "disturbance in self feelings or in the stability of their self image" (Singer 1977b, 471). Psychoanalyst Harry Guntrip commented on this emerging problem of selfhood among many patients: "They are the people who have deep-seated doubts about the reality and viability of their very 'self,' who are ultimately found to be suffering from various degrees of depersonalization, unreality, the dread feeling of 'not belonging,' of being fundamentally isolated and out of touch with the world. . . . The problem here is not relations with other people, but whether one is or has a self" (Guntrip, quoted in Frosh 1987, 249).

In *New Maladies of the Soul*, Kristeva (1995) considers the ques-tion of whether it is possible to speak of a new type of analysand, whose problems correspond to the contradictions of modern life. This new pa-tient, she notes, is "living in a piecemeal and accelerated space and time," and, "left without a sexual, subjective, or moral identity, this amphibian is a being of boundaries, a borderline, or a 'false self'—a body that acts, often without even the joys of such performative drunken-ness" (7). She describes in this patient a "difficulty in expressing one-self, and a general malaise caused by a language experienced as 'artificial,' 'empty,' or 'mechanical.'" (9). Kristeva notes the need for new categories to describe these patients, "new classification systems that take into account wounded 'narcissism,' 'false personalities,' 'borderline states,' and 'psychosomatic conditions'" (9).

These observations of a new type of analysand raise the question of whether this reflects the emergence of new conditions in individu-als, possibly in response to new social conditions or instead, reflects theoretical changes in psychoanalysis. Kristeva poses this question: "Have patients changed or has analytic practice changed, such that ana-lysts have sharpened their interpretations of previously neglected symp-tomatologies?" (9).

One important theoretical shift in psychoanalysis that contributed to the recognition of these self disorders was the emergence of a new theoretical vocabulary that signaled a paradigm shift in psychoanalytic theory, from one centered on the Oedipus Complex to one centered on problems of narcissism from the pre-oedipal period. As Jessica Benjamin puts it, "Narcissus rivals Oedipus as the dominant metaphor of contemporary psychoanalysis. Analysts no longer focus exclusively on the instinctual conflicts that develop through the triangular relationship of child and parents, the Oedipus complex. Now pathologies of the self, or narcissistic disorders, are at least of equal importance in psychoanalytic practice and discussion" (Benjamin 1988, 137).

This paradigm shift is one that replaces the Freudian concern with oedipal conflicts involving the relation between individual instincts and a prohibitive and regulatory culture, with a focus on the development of a sense of self within the context of mother-infant relations. This shift occurs with the rise to prominence of the school of psychoanalysis known as object relations theory, with its emphasis on how persons construct selves in early infancy through relationship to the parents, especially the mother.

While the term "object relations" is used in varying contexts to refer to various theorists or groups of theorists, it is broadly defined as a focus on interactions with external and internal (real and imagined) "objects" or others, and on the relationship between their internal and external object worlds (Greenberg and Mitchell 1983, 14). The shift, which Greenberg and Mitchell term the shift from the "drive" model to the "relational" model, entails the incorporation into the theory of the fundamental importance of the object or other toward which the child is oriented and from which the child incorporates the emotional and cognitive material out of which a sense of self is built. The attention to object relations entails a widening of focus from an isolated individual invested with "wishes" to encompass the presence and adequacy of others, most often the mother, who gratifies these wishes (Mitchell 1988). Object relations theorists explore the process of the infant's attachment to, and differentiation from, the mother, and identify the effects of traumas or disappointments occurring at this early pre-oedipal stage (from age two months to five years). In this stage, the relationship between mother and child becomes the matrix out of which a self is constructed—a self with more or less permanent, deeply ingrained patterns of interacting with others. Thus, these early relationships with parents, and particularly the mother, are understood to be the major sources of borderline pathology. Pre-oedipal conflicts, then, became the primary theoretical lens through which particularly disturbed patients were interpreted.

Gender and Cultural Analyses of Self Pathology

In addition to the theoretical shift toward the pre-oedipal construction of self, other observers argue that patients themselves have changed, in response to new social conditions. Many have noted that the appearance of this fragmented and unstable patient is a sign of a more fluid, uncertain, and changing society, thus making borderline personality a "metaphor for an unstable society" (Millon 1987; Paris 1991; Sass 1982). As Sass writes, "Just as the hysterical neurotic of Freud's time—plagued by conflicts of conscience and desire—exemplified the repressive Western culture at the turn of the century, so certain disturbances in an individual's sense of identity and difficulties in maintaining stable human relationships—characteristics attributed to the borderline personality—may reflect the fragmentation of contemporary society" (Sass 1982, 12). Stephen Frosh has shown how modern and postmodern cultural forms contribute to subjective destabilization in an increasingly unstable society. Arguing that the only stable feature of modernity is instability, Frosh maintains that the emergence of the self disorders is a sign that this cultural instability has its psychic and collective costs (Frosh 1991).

Psychologist Theodore Millon attributes the psychic breakdown that borderline disorder represents to an erosion of society: "Where a society's values and practices are fluid and inconsistent, so too will its residents evolve deficits in psychic solidity and stability" (Millon 1987, 363). Millon points to a number of trends in the direction of cultural erosion of stable norms and role models, such as radical changes in family structure due to divorce, coupled with the effects of television, mind-blurring drugs, and the erosion of reparative and cohering social customs and institutions, such as those found among "extended families, church leaders, schoolteachers, and neighbors" (366). Without such structures, children face only a confusing world of shifting values and are thus unable to develop selves: "Scattered and unguided, they are unable to fashion a clear sense of personal identity, a consistent direction for feelings and attitudes, a coherent purpose to existence. They become 'other-directed' persons who vacillate at every turn, overly responsive to fleeting stimuli, shifting from one erratic course to another" (366).

Joel Paris builds on Millon's earlier analysis to argue that rapid social change or "disintegration" is associated with the incidence of borderline personality disorder, as it is expressed behaviorally in "para-suicide," or attempted suicide, a common feature of borderline personality disorder. Relying on Millon's analysis that "the breakdown of social cohesion, of norms, and of families [leads to] the increasing incidence of impulsive behavior, including para-suicide, substance abuse, and chaotic interpersonal relationships," (Paris 1991, 32), Paris extrapolates Millon's argument, pointing to the lack of clear norms, ambiguous and unclear role prescriptions, and narrowing of social supports within contemporary culture, in which the nuclear or single-parent family is the basic social unit. He contrasts this contemporary picture with that of an earlier era when the extended family offered a "larger variety of family ties and social supports." Thus, Paris writes, "Such a model predicts that syndromes such as borderline personality emerge when cultures change too rapidly, leaving behind those without adaptive skills" (33).

The highlighting of social transformations and of the rapidly changing, unstable character of the contemporary cultural experience is important in the analysis of the cultural roots of the self disorders. The appearance of such broad discussions is one indication that the perception of an increase in the self disorders, particularly in borderline personality disorder, has led to the recognition that these disorders might be socioculturally determined.

Yet none of these cultural analyses discusses gender as one of those salient cultural dimensions. This is evident even in those studies of borderline personality disorder in which the predominance of women so diagnosed is explicitly acknowledged. Paris notes almost in passing that borderline personality disorder is "most common among young females and tends to 'burn out' with age" (30). But Paris does not take up the gender theme, moving instead to issues of age as a factor in borderline phenomena.

A more recent cultural analysis of borderline disorder by anthropologist Larry G. Peters gives only slightly more attention to the issue of gender. Peters notes that borderline symptoms of para-suicide or self-mutilation, transient states of numbness or emptiness (dissociation, or a temporary state of altered consciousness), and associated behaviors, such as substance abuse and eating disorders, are "replete with cultural meaning" (Peters 1994, 7). He argues that they are attempts at self-healing in a culture without spiritual guides or community rituals for collective healing. "Through myth and rite, we learn of our identity and bring value to the world. The lack of sacred myth and rites in our culture has led to an erosion of meaning for both sexes. In the extreme, this 'identity diffusion,' i.e., the lack of the goals and values that form personality and community solidarity, is a principal feature in Borderline Personality Disorder" (7).

Peters notes the predominance of women among those exhibiting the behaviors associated with the borderline syndrome. He states that Western cultural pressures may be responsible for some of these behaviors, such as the pressures for women to be thin, which contributes to eating disorders. Yet, more generally, he states, borderline personality disorder may reflect "Western feminine social reality"; and, drawing on Phyllis Chesler, he writes that it may function as "a mirror image of the feminine social experience and the penalty for being feminine" (5).

Yet while calling attention to the women-specific issues pertinent to the borderline syndrome, Peters moves away from this specificity and does not develop the cultural gender analysis of borderline syndrome that is so provocatively suggested by his analysis.

On one hand, then, these cultural analyses draw our attention to important historical and social transformations affecting individuals' construction of self. However, the gender asymmetry of the disorders of the self poses a challenge to these cultural accounts. The predominance of women among those receiving the diagnosis of borderline calls for further analysis.

The Regime of the Self

From a more sociohistorical perspective, the shift in vocabulary toward self and the appearance of crises of selfhood can be discerned as part of a wider proliferation of discourses and practices of selfhood that Nikolas Rose, drawing on Foucault and Deleuze and Guattari, terms the "regime of self" (Rose 1996). The psychological disciplines and practices are central to this regime of the self, operating to perpetuate the self as a "regulative ideal" through which persons are defined as "individuals inhabited by an inner psychology that animates and explains our conduct and strives for self-realization, self-esteem, and self-fulfillment in everyday life" (3). From this point of view, what we conceive of as the "self" is a historical invention rather than an ontological fact, and this idea of self becomes a regulative norm against which unstable selves are measured.

Rose locates this regulative ideal in a larger process of what Foucault called "subjectification," made up of "regimes of knowledge through which human beings have come to recognize themselves as certain kinds of creature, the strategies of regulation and tactics of action to which these regimes of knowledge have been connected, and the correlative relations that human beings have established with themselves, in taking themselves as subjects" (11).

Rose emphasizes that this is not simply a shift in language, but is bound up in a set of institutions and practices that he terms, following Deleuze and Guattari, the "assemblage": "Subjectification is not to be understood by locating it in a universe of meaning or an interactional context of narratives, but in a complex of apparatuses, practices, machinations, and assemblages within which human being has been fabricated, and which presuppose and enjoin particular relations with ourselves" (10). This broader institutional context of language led Deleuze and Guattari to draw on Foucault's concept of the "enunciative modality" to speak of "assemblages of enunciation," which governs the times and spaces of language: "Who can speak? From where can they speak? What relations are in play between the person who is speaking and the object of which they speak, and those who are the subjects of their speech?" (174).

In order to situate borderline discourse within a larger process of subjectification, we must understand such discourses within the context of the institutional practices and power relations of psychiatry. Thus while this study focuses on discourse, language, and narrative as it is negotiated between client and therapist, it is also important to situate these relations within an institutional context that includes professional organizations and journals, medical and psychiatric hospitals, and pharmaceutical corporations. Together, these institutions constitute what Ingleby called the "psy complex" (Ingleby 1985) and that Rose simply terms "psy." The psy complex is important in two senses. First, a crucial aspect of this psy complex is the dissemination of professional clinical theories, case analyses, and clinical descriptions. These texts form the objectified knowledge (Smith 1990) that psychiatrists draw upon in their interpretation of borderline patients. It is important to emphasize that such objectified knowledge mediates the relation between the therapist as knower and the borderline patient. Particular assumptions regarding the contours of selfhood and the signs and symptoms of underlying mental disorders act as an interpretive lens through which particular women patients are seen and understood. When the language describing mental disorder is pejorative, as it frequently is even in official definitions of borderline personality disorder (Linehan 1993, 16–18) or when the label "borderline" is used in pejorative ways (Reiser and Levenson 1984), this lays the groundwork for a view of patients that is critical of women rather than compassionate toward them (Becker 1997).

Second, beyond the texts of objectified knowledge, the psy complex structures the relations between women patients and psychiatric professionals. The narratives that emerge from the psychotherapeutic encounter, in other words, are located in particular power relations between therapist and patient, an organization of power and knowledge, which "grant powers to some and delimit the powers of others, enable some to judge and some to be judged, some to cure and some to be cured, some to speak truth and others to acknowledge its authority and embrace it, aspire to it, or submit to it" (Rose 1996, 175).

Narrative Analysis: Texts and Social Contexts

Recent interdisciplinary work in interpretive social analysis has brought narrative to the foreground of social life (Bruner 1987; Gergen 1991; Herman 1999; Maines 1993; Polkinghorne 1988; Richardson 1995). Narrative, as Herman points out, is a creative cultural technology of power and knowledge that conjures an imaginary version of the world, giving form and shape to social reality (Herman 1999, 53). Far from transparently describing past events, narratives are themselves significant social acts that produce meaning through devices such as characterization, temporal ordering, and plot structure (Bruner 1987; Maines 1993).

Narrative, then, as Laurel Richardson writes, is "both a mode of reasoning and a mode of representation. People can 'apprehend' the world narratively and people can 'tell' about the world narratively" (Richardson 1995, 200). Richardson cites Jerome Bruner's positing of the narrative mode of reasoning as a major alternative to the logicodeductive mode.

As a text produced through the interaction between patient and clinician, the clinical case narrative can be conceptualized as a story produced jointly by patient and therapist. In this way, case narratives can be considered to be coauthored: "The case study . . . may be seen as a kind of text, constructed jointly by clinician and client" (Gelfond 1991, 247). Clients seeking treatment play a role in the production of meaning in the case narrative. From this perspective, women deemed borderline are not passive victims of a monolithic psychiatric establishment, but rather are active negotiators of the meanings of their psychic and bodily distress.

Yet, as Gergen and Kaye point out, clinical case narratives tend to be more reflective of the therapist's own theoretical frameworks than of the patient's perspective, because the process of therapy is one of replacing the patient's narrative with that of the therapist (Gergen and Kaye 1992). Narratives are, in the modernist scheme, meant to reflect reality accurately. The therapist's reality is viewed as more accurate than the client's, and thus, therapy results in the gradual replacement of the client's own story with the therapist's narrative. And while the patients' narrative is potentially under suspicion as being either inaccurate, or at the very least, an ineffective blueprint for living, the therapist's narrative never comes under the same scrutiny. Thus "the client's narrative is either destroyed or incorporated—but in any case replaced—by the professional account" (169).

A central aspect of the construction of the professional account of any disorder is a formal interpretation of the origins or causes of the patient's symptoms. In its orientation toward origins, the clinical case narrative, Peter Brooks points out, resembles in form and intention the detective story, "which claims that all action is motivated, causally

enchained, and eventually comprehensive as such to the perceptive observer" (Brooks 1984, 269). "Faced with fragmentary evidence, clues
scattered within present reality, he who would explain must reach back
to a story in the past which accounts for how the present took on its
configuration" (270). The case narrative, Brooks argues, is like the detective story in that each is a search for the origins of the present mystery. For the borderline case narratives, the origin is sought in early
childhood, and in particular, in the formation of the self and any de-
viations in that process.

Yet Brooks's analogy points to another similarity between the clinical
case narrative and the detective story: Each uses fictional strategies of
storytelling to convey meaning. A case history by Freud, for example, is
"radically allied to the fictional since its causes and connections depend on probabilistic constructions rather than authoritative facts" (284).

Freud himself, of course, had noted early on in his writings with
Breuer, *Studies in Hysteria*, that having been trained as neuropatholo-
gist, he thought it "strange that the case histories I write should read
like short stories and that as one might say, they lack the serious stamp
of science" (Freud, in Marcus 1985, 91). Freud attributes this need for
this fictional style of writing to the nature of the subject itself, hysteria: "I must console myself with the reflection that the nature of the
subject is evidently responsible for this, rather than any preference of
my own." Stephen Marcus argues that Freud's acknowledgment of the
narrative strategies he is obliged to use in his case histories carried over
to his view of the aim of psychoanalysis:

> In the course of psychoanalytic treatment, nothing less than
> "reality" itself is made, constructed, or reconstructed. A
> complete story—"intelligible, consistent, and unbroken"—is
> the theoretical, created end story. It is a story, or a fiction, not
> only because it has a narrative structure but also because the
> narrative account has been rendered in language, in conscious
> speech, and no longer exists in the deformed language of
> symptoms, the untranslated speech of the body. At the end—at
> the successful end—one has come into possession of one's own
> story. (Marcus 1985, 71–72)

More recently, psychoanalysis has drawn on a conception of narrative construction to understand the practices of psychoanalytic therapy and interpretation (Hoffman 1991; Lesser 1996; Schafer 1989; Spence 1984). In a review of these developments, Louis Sass notes that narrative or "social constructionist" analysts call attention to the "fictive devices" of their practices, beginning with a critique of the realistic commitment to certain basic narratives that are taken as referents for reality, including past childhood memories and psychic structures (Sass 1994). The critics of psychotherapy, writes Sass, "have challenged these realist assumptions, arguing that psychoanalytic interpretations are less discoveries than creations and that memories are more invented than retrieved" (97). More than simply a deconstructive critique of psychoanalytic practices, however, these moves toward narrative have been embraced as clinical innovations. The narrative psychoanalysts believe that the practice of psychoanalytic interpretation can become more efficacious only with the embrace of invented, rhetorical, and constructionist views. Hence the search for truth or reality is a clinical hindrance to the process, and cramps the aesthetic, creative enterprise. For example, Roy Schafer writes that the task of the analyst is to help analysands become "more versatile, sophisticated, and relativistic historians of their lives" (Schafer, in Sass 1994, 100). Schafer, Sass observes, "stresses fostering the analysand's self-conscious awareness of the role of his own ongoing interaction in creating an image or conception of the past" (Sass 1994, 100).

If narrative is the central process of psychoanalysis, this sheds light on the difficulties analysts have with borderline patients. Borderline patients give occasion for narrative, yet disrupt that process through either their inability or resistance to give a coherent story or accounting of their lives. Thus, the authors of the borderline case narrative face an interpretational problem: How are the disparate actions of an unstable person understood, rendered intelligible or comprehensible, within the terms of existing psychiatric frames and categories? One way in which this is rhetorically accomplished is to define incomprehensible stories or resistant actions in therapy as signs of an underlying borderline pathology, which is then taken to be the causal agent and the origin of the unpredictable behavior of certain patients. When aspects of the patient's self-presentation do not cohere, or appear to be "off center," this incoherence can be made meaningful by viewing these aspects as the outward expressions of an inner structural disturbance of the self. The narrative of pathology, it could be said, gives the patient (and the analysts) a "fictional coherence" (Moi 1985, 187).

The Web of Narration: Telling Selves

If narratives are constitutive of psychiatric knowledge, narrative is also the fundamental process through which the self is constructed (Bruner 1987; Gergen 1991; Maines 1993). As Jerome Bruner writes, "the self-abstracted person . . . is one who has acquired a biography and can tell his or her life story" (Bruner 1987, 23). The self, as Roy Schafer writes, is a narrative self, and it exists in the telling: "One can only tell a self or encounter it as something told . . . or, as the case may be, tell more than one self. The so-called self exists in versions, only in versions, and commonly in multiple simultaneous versions" (Schafer 1989, 158). As this statement makes clear, Schafer's conception of multiple versions undermines the unitary self that, Rose argues, operates as a "regulatory ideal": "There is nothing here to support the common illusion that there is a single self-entity that each person has and experiences, a self-entity that is, so to speak, out there in nature where it can be objectively (introspectively) observed, clinically analyzed, and then summarized and bound in a technical definition" (158).

If the self is constructed as a fictive coherence, this poses a challenge to a positivist or objectivist view of the self as an inner structure. Jane Flax argues that it is important to recognize when psychoanalysts draw on the objectivist view of the self, a view that is inscribed in the theoretical narratives of what are assumed to be "normal" processes of individual self-development. These "lines of development," Flax points out, posit a linear progression of self-development, which is said to occur in predictable stages from an original primary symbiosis with the mother, through separation and autonomy (Flax 1996). Deviation from these lines, as Flax notes, is understood to contribute to pathology. Flax argues that these developmental stories minimize social influences on subjectivity and identity: "The appearance of essential, teleological processes should be investigated and treated as consequences of social interventions and discursive constructions, not as natural facts." The processes through which the modern subject is constituted as an individual, and our belief in its existence, are historically situated, discourses-dependent, and contingent" (580). The teleology of the self in such developmental lines, moving from fusion to separation and autonomy, reflects the Western valorization of individualism and self-sufficiency, Flax argues. Hence the story of the self is a historical construct, shaped in accord with dominant discourses.

My analysis is based on the guiding assumption that the meaning of the borderline disorder is a rhetorical accomplishment, constructed in the case narrative. This analysis traces the construction of meaning of the disordered self—the self that is disunified, fragmented, unstable, and volatile. I examine the formal interpretation of this unstable self, through a critical investigation of the ways in which psychoanalysts deploy the dominant psychoanalytic narrative of the "normal" self—a self that has proceeded along the normal developmental paths or lines, and whose present manifestation is coherent, unified, and stable.

Another focus of the analysis is the figurative language used to depict the unstable self, including the metaphors and meanings deployed in describing the actions and appearance of the patient deemed borderline. Metaphors, as Laurel Richardson points out, are a constitutive part of language in communicating meaning, creating a description of an idea through comparison or analogy. Further, metaphors communicate cognitive content as well as value commitments (Richardson 1995, 205). In analyzing the language of the case narratives, I focus on how borderline patients' outward appearance, behavior, and subjective states are described through analogy or comparison, exploring the unintended or unconscious cultural and gendered meanings that such comparative descriptions carry. I examine the implications of these metaphorical descriptions for the interpretation of the self. Such metaphors not only reveal unconscious gender assumptions; they also shape analysts' perceptions of borderline women, as well as their subsequent treatment. Hence, they do more than simply describe patients; they contribute to the discourse on borderline patients that shapes how clinicians perceive certain female patients, particularly those who are resistant to therapy or who do not fit existing psychiatric categories.

Narratives of Therapy: Text as Symptom

A central strategy of narrative analysis is to examine "the relationship between texts . . . and their social conditions, both the immediate conditions of the situational context and the more remote conditions of institutional and social structures" (Fairclough 1989, 26). Accounts or narratives of an event are produced in an immediate social relationship between a teller and a listener. Catherine Reissman, in describing her method of analyzing women's and men's narrative accounts of their divorces, writes, "Individuals develop their accounts . . . in interaction with others, both 'real' and imaginary. . . . As a consequence, such accounts are typically co-authored" (Reissman 1990, 16).

The therapeutic relationship is not like one outside the walls of therapy; it is one in which "the patient and the therapist interlock in a curious paradoxical embrace, at once artificial and yet deeply authentic" (Yalom and Elkin 1974, 218). Yalom points out how the structuring of that relationship—in which the patient pays a fee, the hour and time of meeting is fixed, the roles of patient and therapist are not equivalent—makes it an "artificial" social relationship. Yet it is also a highly intimate exchange, and intense reactions may be experienced by patient and therapist.

The terms "transference" and "countertransference" are common parlance in clinical discourse used to refer to the intense, often emotionally charged, reactions of patient and analyst toward one another. These terms refer to Freud's initial discovery that some of his patients showed emotional reactions to him that were rooted in past relationships. Feelings and identifications toward significant others such as parents, in other words, were "transferred" onto Freud himself. "Countertransference" refers to the analyst's own identifications and emotional reactions to the patient. The term "transference" was later broadened to encompass any emotional reaction to the therapist, not necessarily only those rooted in earlier relationships or in childhood conflicts. A patient's transference may be positive, expressed in an idealization of the analyst as an all-giving, omnipotent being, or negative, as revealed in the patient's rage or resistance to the therapy itself. Analysts use an examination of transference as an interpretive device to understand the patient's motives in therapy and to determine the source of the patient's conflicts.

Countertransference is a prominent theme in case narratives of borderline patients, who are renowned for evoking intense reactions in therapists. Commonly referred to as "the difficult patients" in clinical circles, borderline patients appear to place particular demands on therapist's clinical expertise. This turbulent situation forms the social context within which a woman diagnosed as borderline is interpreted within psychiatric discourse, so that the scene of interpretation, in which the meaning of borderline disorder is produced, is not a neutral one. This analysis focuses on how this turbulent situation affects the analytic knowledge produced.

Feminist and literary interpretations of Freud's case narrative of his patient Dora (Freud 1973) examine the implications of countertransference for the ways Freud interprets and narrates Dora's hysteria. Critics have examined the sexual politics of the case by noting that Dora's father had brought his eighteen-year-old daughter to Freud to "bring her to reason" (Freud 1963, 42) in order to minimize the threat she posed to his illicit affair with a family friend, Frau K. Dora also believed that her father had pushed her toward Frau K.'s husband in exchange for her keeping the affair secret. As Kahane notes, one strategy these critics use is to reverse Freud's question regarding Dora's transference: What did Dora want of Freud? What unconscious desires and past relationships was she projecting onto Freud, that might be a source of her resistance to the analysis and to Freud's interpretations? Feminist critics reverse this question: What did Freud want from Dora? What were Freud's unconsciously repressed desires and motives that shaped his perceptions of Dora? (Kahane 1985, 24) Countertransference draws attention to Freud's assumptions about femininity and female desire— inevitably derived from cultural norms and constitutive of gender ideology. Some feminist critics have faulted Freud for his insistence that Dora accept as normal a sexual desire for her father's friend who had tried to seduce her (Ramas 1985; Showalter 1985). Showalter comments, "Freud failed Dora because he was too quick to impose his own language on her mute communications. His insistence on the sexual origins of hysteria blinded him to the social factors contributing to it" (Showalter 1985,160).

Others have pointed out how Freud's epistemological aims affect his narrative (Marcus 1985; Moi 1985). Toril Moi has focused on the case as a power struggle between two models of knowledge, set up as opposing epistemologies by the terms of patriarchal bourgeois scientific ideals: on one hand, Freud's desire for knowledge as complete, unitary, with nothing missing; and on the other hand, Freud's construction of Dora's knowledge as fragmented, incomplete, a feminine "tale" based on gossip. Dora's narrative is presented in Freud's text as appearing to him in a form that "cannot be conceptualized as a whole; it is dispersed and has been assembled piecemeal from feminine sources" (Moi 1985, 196).

Yet as Moi points out, Freud's aim of "complete elucidation" of all the mysteries of Dora's case rests in uneasy tension with a persistent doubt and anxiety about its fragmentary and incomplete character. "His prefatory remarks oscillate constantly between the theme of fragmentation and the notion of totality" (185). For example, Freud writes of his decision to call the case a "fragment" for several reasons: Dora broke off treatment prematurely and thus left Freud with an incomplete analysis; the text itself is assembled from Freud's fragmentary notes and the reconstruction of his memories of the details of the case; only the results of the case are presented without interpretation; the case itself is but a fragment of many cases of hysteria and thus provides only a partial picture of the workings of hysteria. Overall, the political significance of the case, argues Moi, is that it is an example of "phallocentric" epistemology, which constructs its own binary oppositions between totality and completeness, and inferior mutilated fragments; between this ideal of wholeness and its negative underside—the fragment; and the assignment, within contemporary Western representational systems, of gendered connotations to this duality. The masculine is associated with the ideal, and the feminine is associated with the incomplete, piecemeal, and fragmentary remains. "Nowhere is patriarchal ideology to be seen more clearly than in the definition of the feminine as the negative of the masculine and this is precisely how Freud defines Dora and the 'feminine' epistemology she is supposed to represent" (198). Moi's analysis suggests that Freud's epistemology, in practice, resembles in spite of his efforts at the elimination of holes, Derrida's notion of *différance*: "The fragment depends on the supplement, which depends on other fragments depending on other supplements, and so on ad infinitum" (187).

While perhaps reductive of the complexities of Freud's narrative, Moi's analysis alerts us to the relations among desire, power, and knowledge in narrativity. Significantly, this desire is forged in the insecurity of Freud's interactions with a female patient who resists Freud's interpretation of the story, to the point of abruptly terminating her treatment with him. Yet he may recover from this rejection, suggests Moi, through the narrative itself. "When Dora dismisses Freud like a servant, she paradoxically rescues him from further epistemological insecurity. He is left, then, the master of the writing of Dora" (197).

As Moi's analysis illustrates, a critical concern with the transferential dynamics of narrative is not narrowly focused on a particular author's private personal feelings, which may be said to bias his/her perception of a patient. Rather, they refer to the ways that perceptions and feelings themselves are structured, or as James Clifford states, "overdetermined," by "forces ultimately beyond the control either of an author or an interpretive community. These contingencies—of language, rhetoric, power, and history—must now be openly confronted in the process of writing" (Clifford 1986, 25). Transference, then, within the critical analyses of Freudian narratives, refers to the way "knowing" is embodied, rooted in, and channeled through desires of which the knower may not be aware; and in turn, to the way desires are structured by historical relations of power, of which gender is one of the most central.

The text, then, is produced in this unique and paradoxical relationship, marked by currents of desire and conflict. The relations between analyst and analysand become the conditions for the production of the textual narrative of the patient's life and treatment history. The clinical case account is thus not only a psychiatric-medical story of a particular patient, but also a record of the treatment situation and of the interaction between psychiatrist and patient. The text thus is symptomatic of the power and transferential relations of the psychoanalytic situation.

The Gender Context

The second level of social context within which the text is situated consists of the "more remote conditions of institutional and historical structures" (Fairclough 1989, 26). The production of a narrative, in other words— the relationship of telling and listening—is itself situated in, and depends on, wider historical and social contexts. The meanings produced in the narrative are drawn from that wider context. Reissman writes, "Meanings are not only a private construction, but have a collective counterpart, representing history and cultural understandings. . . . [Texts] are also co-authored in a more general sense because they depend on consensual [or contested] meanings, just as they rely on historically situated motives" (Reissman 1990, 13, 16).

The psychiatrist-patient dyad, then, is situated in the wider institutional and cultural contexts of scientific power, which in turn are embedded in cultural understandings of gender, which provide psychiatrists with the "historically situated motives" or meanings for the analysis of female patients. In the psychiatric and scientific interpretation of the female malady, as feminist writers have pointed out, dominant images of women that are specific to the prevailing ideological construction of gender figure heavily in such psychiatric or medical constructions of the female patient. Dominant images of the feminine body and mind, whether viewed as the site of reproductive order and disorder, as in the nineteenth-century hysterical body, or as the site of discipline and control, as in the twentieth-century anorexic body, shape the medical construction of feminine disorder.

Another Story: Symptom as Text

Jane Ussher has argued for the importance of keeping the psychic distress of women in mind in feminist deconstructions of the categories of madness. Thus, while a major aspect of my analysis concerns how women deemed borderline are represented as disordered personalities—linguistically and narratively—it is not possible to dismiss women's suffering as a mere chimera of psychiatric discourse. The borderline case narratives offer a window into some troubling and complex forms of psychic suffering, and part of my aim is to situate this suffering within gender relations and meanings in order to gain an understanding of their gendered dimensions and cultural sources.

This does not mean, however, that we are able to gain access to women's madness as a real, unmediated experience, outside the frameworks of language through which we come to perceive them. As Ussher notes, women's own experience and understanding of madness is itself constituted through those dominant frameworks. "The individual in distress, a distress that is undoubtedly real in the sense that she is really suffering, experiences that distress in a way which is defined by the particular discourse associated with madness" (Ussher 1992, 12). Thus it is important to avoid the tendency to view the descriptions of borderline disorder, whether given by analysts or by women themselves, as an unmediated window into the real. Madness, no less than any other phenomenon, is a matter of representation, and a case narrative of a woman diagnosed as borderline is told through the frameworks of knowledge and power through which psychiatric categories attain their institutional existence.

My strategy is to put into question or bracket the label and construct of "borderline" as a unitary phenomenon, an inner diathesis, and to consider the potential social sources of the particular symptoms women bring to the therapeutic encounter. Thus I consider these symptoms as discursively produced in the text, but also produced in women as responses to social conditions, intelligible in a broader context of gender and power in late modern society. Hence I am concerned with the negotiation of meaning of women's experience in the context of discursive frameworks of psychiatric/psychoanalytic knowledge and power. My analysis is thus an "attempt to reflexively map multiple discourses that occur in a given social space" (Denzin 1997, xvii).

My aim is to "deconstruct meaning claims in order to look for the modes of power they carry and to force open a space for the emergence of counter-meanings" (Ferguson 1991, 323). The goal is to deconstruct what is audible in the text, in order to hear what is inaudible: women's symptomatic body. What is it saying, and how might we read or hear this body culturally? As Dana Becker writes of borderline symptoms in women, "The distress is real; the diagnosis is a fiction that has become a fact of psychiatric classification. If we follow the evolution of borderline concept to borderline diagnosis, the fictive nature of the diagnosis becomes yet more clear and the question of the origin and nature of the distress we now term borderline becomes more pressing" (Becker 1997, 48).

In framing women's symptoms in this way, I draw on feminist analyses of women's madness as a form of resistance to the conditions of their lives (Bordo 1993; Ong 1988). In her analysis of the episodes of spirit possession in young Malaysian factory workers, Ong argues that the spirit attacks, which were interpreted as hysteria by Western medical authorities, could be read as the young women's unconscious resistance to the constraints of their social role, as well as to the rigors of factory life. "Young, unmarried women in Malay society are expected to be shy, obedient, and deferential, to be observed and not heard. In spirit possession episodes, they speak in other voices that refuse to be silenced" (Ong 1988, 33)

In her analysis of "female maladies" such as hysteria, agoraphobia, and anorexia, Bordo suggests that the symptoms of these disorders may be read as "literalizations" of women's social situation. For Bordo, the symptoms of these female maladies are politically symbolic: "The symptomatology of these disorders reveals itself as textuality. Loss of mobility, loss of voice, inability to leave the home, feeding others while starving self, taking up space and whittling down the space one's body takes up—all have symbolic meaning, all have political meaning within the varying rules governing the historical construction of gender" (Bordo 1993, 168). Bordo argues that these women can be viewed as unconsciously protesting the constraints of gender roles through their bodies, rather than through verbal articulation. Their bodily symptoms, therefore, can be read as signs of women's subjectivity and social position. "In hysteria, agoraphobia, and anorexia, the woman's body may thus be viewed as a surface on which conventional constructions of femininity are exposed starkly to view, through their inscription in extreme or hyperliteral form" (175).

Robert Romanyshyn also provides a perspective for an interpretive reading of symptoms as signs of culturally excluded meanings. Symptoms are carriers of meanings that the dominant culture would deny or repress. Symptoms are a way of both concealing and preserving a cultural situation; "to be sure, a symptom as a way of ignoring or forgetting something is also a way of preserving or remembering it" (Romanyshyn 1989, 13). Symptoms are shadows, traces of what the dominant culture, particularly its configuration of embodied experience, excludes. Symptoms may therefore carry important meaning as signs of a gap between a given cultural order—the dominant assumed categories for experience—and the actual ways people experience their bodies: "In every symptom there is, so to speak, the whisper of a direction, the hint of a path about how one can find one's way back to health or balance or, perhaps most descriptively, home. Symptoms are a memory of this path, this way home, this way back to what has been forgotten, lost, ignored, or otherwise left behind" (13). "The shadow as carrier of what we would deny demands our recognition and attention, and if it is ignored or too easily dismissed it returns, perhaps in an even more intense fashion" (163).

In *Becoming Woman* (1997), Camilla Griggers analyzes the "politics of memory and affect" embedded in the symptomatic breakdown of women in postmodern society, arguing that it is an exaggerated sign of a more general breakdown in the social body. Griggers notes the "dilemma of (mal)adaptation and (dys)function as paradigmatic of the state of being feminine in postmodern culture . . . femininity becomes disordered if not pathological in order to adapt to a pathological and disordered socialization" (110). Drawing on Deleuze and Guattari, Griggers defines the feminine subject as an "abstract-machine," a "conceptual formation that, when activated, legitimizes . . . an overcoding of signifiers and meanings" (x). Women's bodies and nervous systems are linked to the social body and thus become carriers for social violence. Symptomatic acting-out, states of dissociation, self-mutilation, and anorexia become signs of that systemic social violence:

> While the breakdown is represented in our culture as an event occurring within the individual, nowhere is the abstract social organization of the feminine more apparent than in the moment of its breakdown. A daunting creature when all her systems run, she is a hyperthymic overachiever, technologically loaded with electronic-prosthetic memory, neurochemical-prosthetic personality, and media-prosthetic desires. But breakdowns are common, and when they happen, one can glimpse the (dys)functional organs ordering her as a feminine social subject. She typically drives too fast while complaining of being driven, consumes too much while rushing to the toilet to throw up. Sometimes she acts out. Often she is chronically 'depressed,' not to mention psychoneurologically wired for psychosis. (106)

Describing the recent surge in feminine disorders such as post-traumatic stress disorder, anorexia-bulimia, and borderline personality disorder, Griggers reads them as exaggerated signs of a more widespread social dysfunction:

> Femininity as a cultural category is constituted partly as a potentiality for receiving and signing the flow of social violences, that the feminine position is constituted as such within a nervous system producing women as victims/survivors, self-mutilators, dysfunctionals, and designated crazies. Within that ground of being, to adapt (to not suicide) is to (mal)adapt. (110)

Griggers focuses in particular on dissociation, a common symptom of post-traumatic stress disorder, multiple personality disorder, and borderline personality disorder. Dissociation is a defense mechanism, a state of altered consciousness in which painful memories are split off and repressed, resulting in a fragmentation of subjectivity. For Griggers, dissociation in women signifies not simply individual women's suppressed memories, but the suppression and denial of historical memories of a circulating social violence. The symptomatic resurfacing of these memories in the form of numbness, states of depersonalization, or self-mutilation is frequently managed through psychopharmacology, a practice that aids in viewing such symptomatic memories as only individual rather than social in origin. Griggers's cultural analysis helps to reconnect these individual women's symptoms to their social sources.

These cultural feminist and poststructural analyses provide a framework for reading the borderline as a phenomenon with cultural significance. The symptoms that come to be commonly grouped together under the borderline label—fragmented or unstable identity, feelings of emptiness or numbness, depersonalization, self-mutilation—may be meaningfully understood as exaggerated or extreme forms of some of the cultural contradictions of gender in late modern society, as fault lines of a cultural order in which the contradictions are visible in the moment of breakdown of the feminine subject.

Andrew Samuels, in a clinical article on treating borderline patients, writes that the patient deemed borderline holds a fascination. The borderline patient can speak without "completely letting go of being sane," and is thus "not completely crazy, not incapable of making a point or a decision, not dead" (Samuels 1988, 182). Samuels depicts the "ecstasy" of a madness that maintains a grasp on "reality": "intense affect, sometimes with depersonalization; impulsive behavior, sometimes directed against the self, brief psychotic experiences; disturbed personal relationships, sometimes exceedingly intimate and sometimes distant. This could be the profile of a saint" (118).

In my exploration of the case narratives, I'm moved to listen more closely to this purportedly maladjusted woman because of a feminist concern for the limitations and the costs of adjusting in the present society. What does this patient, who is positioned at these borderlines, reveal about the cultural conditions for women's identity and subjectivity, in early-twenty-first-century society? How thin is the borderline between supposedly normal feminine subjecthood in postmodern society, and madness? What normal forms of organization ensure women's continued survival within the violence of this cultural order?

The borderline category is also a site of contradictions in psychiatric theory and practice. How does this maladjusted patient, who does not fit existing diagnostic categories, reveal the limitations of those categories? How does her lack of adjustment call into question the authority, the naturalness, of those categories, such that another look is necessary to understand how they came to be constructed in the first place?

From this partial, feminist reading, this book explores this site—the psychiatric borderline text—as a fruitful place of intersections, entanglements, and boundary blurring that may be revealing not only of the working of the construction of psychiatric notions of female personality, but also as the site where women break through the boundaries of normal feminine selfhood—a site where the limitations of those borders (surrounding the construct of "normal femininity") are more visible, and where women's disruptions signal the important effects of these borders. These women are the embodiment of the marginal, yet currently transitional and contradictory position of women in contemporary culture and the costs of that contradictory space.

Overview of the Book

Chapter 2 is devoted to a genealogy of the borderline category within psychiatric discourse. The borderline concept is particularly revealing of the discursive construction of psychiatric categories, and of the process of negotiating the boundaries between sanity and madness. This genealogy of the borderline concept has two main concerns: 1) to deconstruct the borderline category as itself an unstable, ambiguous, and contradictory category that sharply highlights the problematic relations of psychiatric taxonomy to the patients so categorized; and 2) to trace the "feminization" of the diagnosis over time.

Chapter 2 frames the genealogy of the borderline as psychiatry's attempt to discover and represent the ambiguous terrain between sanity and madness, which Martin Leichtman referred to as an "undefined wilderness." I discuss three phases of meaning of the borderline concept: 1) the late nineteenth century and early medical psychiatry's concept of the "borderland"; 2) psychoanalysis in the United States, from 1930 through the 1970s; and 3) biopsychiatry after 1980.

In the first phase, physicians began to recognize some patients who retained their powers of reason, yet nonetheless showed signs of disturbance. Andrew Wynter used the term "borderland" to designate this type of patient. I discuss the use of the borderland concept as a way of categorizing social and moral transgression as "degeneracy," and argue that the borderland concept is a particularly revealing illustration of the impact of social norms and moral codes on how the borders of psychological normality are drawn.

In the second phase, Adolph Stern first described patients occupying the "border line" between neurosis and psychosis. This chapter traces the discourse on this borderline patient within psychoanalytic thought to examine the shift toward focus on the ego, character, and more recently, the self in therapeutic discourse. I also discuss post-Freudian psychoanalytic theories of the borderline category, focusing on object relations theory.

I then move on to a discussion of biopsychiatry beginning in the 1980s, when borderline personality disorder appeared for the first time in the Diagnostic and Statistical Manual of Mental Disorders. Here the chapter moves into a detailed review of the debates and conflicts within psychiatry and between psychiatry and other mental health fields concerning the meaning of the borderline diagnosis and its status as a pejorative label for the troublesome (female) patient. Its meaning remains contested and ambiguous within the mental health field.

Chapter 2 concludes by asserting that in the face of such ambiguity, pejorative connotations, and lack of agreement as to its meaning, the borderline category, like hysteria, refers to multiple conditions. Further, it is open to social and political manipulation as a medical label used to explain and control certain women patients in psychological distress. The chapter closes with a clear statement of the need for further examination of the types of women receiving the diagnosis and the language and theories used to interpret the borderline patient.

Chapter 3 focuses on the theme of instability as it appears in clinical theories and case narratives of patients deemed borderline, and examines the significance of instability to images of femininity in Western culture. First, drawing on the work of Butler, Cixous and Clément, and Irigaray, the chapter outlines a feminist critique of the representation of femininity in Western culture, focusing on the exclusion of feminine difference, and the marginalization of women in the binary logic of gender. I then examine hysteria and its linkages to feminine instability both within psychiatry and in the wider culture.

This review forms the critical context for an examination of the language of instability in the case narratives of borderline patients. I discuss the borderline concept as well as the underlying ideal of stable selfhood that informs the interpretation of the borderline patient, against which the selves of women are measured as unstable. I then discuss the language of unstable selfhood more closely, focusing on the themes of emptiness and fluidity as markers of borderline psychic instability. Illustrative examples of this language are drawn from case studies. Here I consider the cultural associations between fluidity and femininity.

I then discuss the turbulent therapeutic interaction between therapist and patient as the context for the production of the case narrative. Case examples illustrate how psychiatrists view those patients who appear elusive or resistant to analysis as psychologically unstable, and I draw parallels between hysteria and borderline as labels for female resistance. Drawing on the concept of transference, I show how the borderline case texts illustrate how transferential dynamics play a role in shaping the interpretation of the borderline patient.

While women constitute the majority of those diagnosed as borderline, some men also receive this diagnosis. In the last section of chapter

3, therefore, I examine two case narratives of men in order to compare the ways the borderline patient's unstable self is interpreted. The cases of men contrast with those of women, and yet illustrate the ways gender meanings related to masculinity are invoked in the narratives. This emerges either as a depiction of the male borderline patient as "hyper-masculine," or as expressing a failed masculinity that puts the stability of his self in question.

Chapter 4 explores one particular manifestation of instability discussed in the case narratives of women: the theme of fragmented, dual selfhood. I discuss four clinical cases in which such split selfhood is a prominent symptom, and analyze the interpretation of this subjective fragmentation in relation to the representation of women. In these cases, patients are described as manifesting a split between a passive, surface self that is outwardly conforming, and one or more underlying partial selves that conflict with that surface self. From a feminist cultural perspective (and drawing on the work of feminist psychoanalyst Jane Flax and cultural theorist Susan Bordo), it is necessary to read these conflicting selves as representative of contradictory social expectations for women, embedded in the logic of gender and affecting even the lives of women who aren't necessarily defined as "mad," but embodied in particularly graphic form in the minds and bodies of women deemed borderline. The passive surface self conforms to cultural expectations for traditional forms of femininity, and the more autonomous and empowered selves are usually denied expression for women and represent desires that do not conform to traditional feminine norms. Women faced with such contradictory cultural meanings of femininity face a double bind in the construction of subjectivity, creating the conditions for the oscillations of identity expressed in exaggerated form in the patient deemed borderline.

The last part of the chapter examines in depth two autobiographical narratives of women who have been diagnosed with borderline personality disorder. The first is Susanna Kaysen's *Girl, Interrupted* (Kaysen 1993), her memoir of her experience in a mental hospital in 1968, when she was eighteen. The second narrative is Jane Wanklin's autobiographical account *Let Me Make It Good: A Chronicle of My Life with Borderline Personality Disorder* (Wanklin 1997). These autobiographies show us how women deemed borderline in two different eras interpret and narrativize their psychological distress. While Kaysen questions the conventional feminine social roles that she resisted and that confined her, and ultimately challenges the norms of mental health through which she was deemed mad, Wanklin seeks answers for her madness in early childhood abuse. Yet Wanklin's narrative also vividly illustrates the peculiar stresses and contradictions of a consumer-driven and media-saturated culture, stresses that she experiences and expresses through her body in graphic ways.

Chapter 5 focuses on another prominent symptom in cases of women deemed borderline: rage. This chapter shows how psychiatrists interpret women's rage as pathological and how this in turn leads to the definition of women deemed borderline as lacking coherent, rational selves.

This chapter analyzes in depth three cases in which rage dominates the text. I focus on two central narrative devices used by analysts that depoliticize women's rage: 1) the rhetoric of rage as a flood, in which analysts depict rage as an overwhelming, irrational force that is fundamentally separate from the borderline patient's self; and 2) displacement of rage from paternal to maternal sources, in which analysts attribute the sources of rage to early mothering while ignoring its sources in women's social relations in patriarchal culture. These rhetorical strategies render women's rage pathological and medical, thus eliding their political meaning.

Women deemed borderline pose a challenge to the authority of the analyst as knower, and the case texts illustrate the turbulence and conflict that mark the relationship between women and their therapists. Here the concept of transference is particularly useful in showing how therapeutic interactions shape interpretation. The intensity of the anger expressed by the woman deemed borderline destabilizes the analyst's position of authority and thus shapes the direction of the narrative. The context of therapy, then, is not a neutral medium for the objective interpretation of patients' symptoms, but rather a tension-filled emotional field within which analysts and patients struggle over the meaning of women's anger. Here we find another source of the borderline label as a defense against this struggle.

It is important to read women's anger in the context of gender and power, and the cases show how women's rage can be read as resistance to their subordinate position within the culture. Thus, while the split subjectivity discussed in chapter 4 may signify women's embodiment of a cultural double bind, rage may signify the first step toward an active and resistive response to the conditions within which this double bind is created. The book concludes by raising questions regarding the medicalization of women's rage in the context of personality disorders, addressing the relationship between women's resistance and psychiatric interpretation.

Chapter 2

An "Undefined Wilderness"

The History of the Borderline Concept

Our clinical experience tells us that the border of insanity is not a line; it is rather a vast territory with no sharp division: a no-man's-land between sanity and insanity.

(Green 1977, 16)

When we have portrayed the history of the usages of the term "borderline" in psychiatry, we will have simultaneously defined the term. Its history is its meaning.

(Stone, in Cauwels 1992, 361)

Borderline Personality Disorder: A New Female Malady?

DIAGNOSIS, WRITES PHILIP BROWN, is the language of psychiatry, the "social representation of psychiatric knowledge, as well as the psychiatric professions' presentation of self" (Brown 1990, 389). As Brown points out, the critical sociological study of mental illness has focused on the social control functions of psychiatry, yet it has not always recognized that diagnosis has been a central component of this social control. "Giving the name has been the starting point for social labelers. The power to give the name has been a core element in the social control nature of the mental health professions and institutions" (388).

This chapter traces the shifting meanings of the borderline diagnosis. I focus on psychiatry's delineation and conceptualization of the territory that the person diagnosed borderline is said to occupy: the ambiguous, vague, and unstable region between sanity and madness. Psychiatrists in the nineteenth century placed certain persons in this social and taxonomic borderland, situated between socially defined categories of "reason" and "unreason" (Foucault 1965). The way this borderland region is conceptualized has varied considerably over the course of its development, leading to a proliferation of meanings, along with attempts to rid the term of ambiguity and lack of clarity. The term "borderline" has been used in a variety of ways; it has referred to a psychic state, a stage of development, a form of preschizophrenia, an affective disorder, and a personality disorder (Aronson 1985; Meissner 1984).

This diagnosis has been used in multiple ways, as is evident from descriptions of patients diagnosed as borderline. The borderline concept is particularly revealing of the social and discursive construction of psychiatric categories, and of the process of negotiating the boundaries between sanity and madness. This discursive history shows that the depictions and definitions of the borderline disorder refer less to a real underlying mental illness—an identifiable personality disorder—than to changes in psychiatric discourse itself. Further, the borderline category is ambiguous and contradictory, frequently applied to the patient who is socially deviant or marginal. The effect of labeling a patient borderline is to produce a new subject of psychiatry—the unstable inhabitant of the borderland between sanity and madness.

The borderline diagnosis has been feminized over time, and the proportion of women among those diagnosed borderline has grown. Further, some feminist observers have noted that the borderline diagnosis appears to be a contemporary successor to the earlier category of hysteria (Becker 1997; Jimenez 1997). Borderline disorder, like hysteria in the late nineteenth century, is a complex category, describing a markedly diverse range of symptoms, and applied to an increasingly larger number of women who display what is perceived as disturbed or excessive behavior. This chapter pays particular attention to the conceptual threads that contribute to the feminization of the diagnosis.

The changing meanings and uses of the symbolic mobility of the borderline category can be traced through psychiatric discourse. The meaning of "borderline" has changed considerably within psychoanalytic psychiatry since Adolph Stern's initial article in 1938, so much so that, as Becker writes, "the originator of the term would likely not recognize it in its present form" (Becker 1997, xxiii).

Another important conceptual thread traced here is the association of the disorder with the unstable self. My particular focus is on the relationships among conceptions of selfhood, femininity, and madness, and thus I trace the role of the concept of the disturbed, dysfunctional, or fragmented self in the discourse on borderline disorder. If the prominence of the self disorders is part of the contemporary "regime of the self," it is important to examine how the concept of the coherent, unified self, as a regulatory ideal, operates in borderline disorder, particularly for women.

Feminist analyses of women and psychiatry have shown that psychiatric discourse is one of the means by which women are represented as Other to the dominant conceptions of a purportedly rational human subject (Astbury 1996; Showalter 1985; Ussher 1992). Feminine difference, be it biological or psychological, is pathologized as unstable when it is judged against this rational norm. In this sense, social marginality and difference are related to perceptions of psychological instability. The borderline is a category entangled with notions of social deviance and difference. This chapter traces that entanglement.

The contemporary definition of the borderline diagnosis appears in the fourth and latest edition of the Diagnostic and Statistical Manual of Mental Disorders, or DSM-IV. The current definition is little changed from the first entry into the DSM in 1980, and can be said to represent a codification of the definition of the disorder.

Yet in spite of its codification within official diagnostic classification, the meaning of the borderline concept has remained ambiguous and controversial. Like hysteria, borderline is a broad category, which includes a wide array of symptoms that are open to multiple interpretations. One commentator calls the multiple meanings "both bewildering and irreconcilable" and recommends that the term be dropped from psychiatric classification (Aronson 1985). This ambiguity is reflected in its history, as from the beginning psychiatrists grappling with the meaning of the borderline, in their attempts to treat particularly difficult patients, offered widely divergent definitions. With no firm object behind the proliferating definitions, the term's meanings are shifting and uncertain. Behind the borderline category, in other words, lies not a "real," unified disorder that is constant through time, but rather, a complex, fragmented, and shifting history of psychiatric discourse and institutional practices.

In the face of such semantic ambiguity and categorical uncertainty, the question of borderline disorder as a new "female malady"—or more generally, the relationship between gender and the borderline diagnosis—requires careful scrutiny. Explaining the predominance of women among those diagnosed as borderline requires an investigation of the conceptual history of this term to examine how this unstable category became associated with women.

My analysis draws from Foucault's method of "genealogy" to trace these changing meanings of the borderline construct. Foucault writes, "If the genealogist listens to history, [s]he finds that there is 'something altogether different' behind things: not a timeless and essential secret, but the secret that they have no essence or that their essence was fabricated in a piecemeal fashion from alien forms" (Foucault 1984, 78). Foucault's statement implies an assumption about the nature of "things" such as madness, an assumption crucial to my analysis of the borderline construct: Madness has no underlying unity, as a discrete, definable object with clear boundaries that one can isolate, study, and describe. Rather, the shifting definitions of madness operate to constitute it in a particular way. The discourse constitutes madness as an object. As Bryan Turner writes, "It is the discourse of insanity within the medical profession itself which creates and constitutes a unity which we then call sane and insane behavior. In short, scientific concepts are not neutral descriptions of patterns of behavior, but on the contrary they produce through discursive activity the behavior which they seek to describe" (Turner 1987, 61).

Thus this genealogy does not presume that a phenomenon called "borderline" was already there, prior to the discursive construction of the category, and able to be traced back to its origins. That would be akin to a search for the truth of the borderline as an attempt to "capture the exact essence of things, their purest possibilities, and their carefully protected identities." (Foucault 1984, 78). Nor does it presume that knowledge about borderline disorder evolved in a linear progression, as the outcome of steadily uncovering the "truth" of the phenomenon. Rather, my genealogical analysis presumes that the present meaning of the concept arises from complex and shifting layers of discourse. It presumes that the borderline category is, as Foucault writes, an "unstable assemblage of faults, fissures, and heterogeneous layers that threaten the fragile inheritor from within or from underneath" (82).

Thus, my intent here is not to provide a comprehensive history of the borderline disorder; nor do I give a full discussion of the many different theoretical elaborations on the concept. Rather, I trace some of the conceptual threads that come together to produce the contemporary meaning of the borderline. These conceptual threads shape and construct the idea of the borderline; behind the term, then, is a complex confluence of discursive and social threads, rather than a unified entity that we might discover.

Further, this genealogy is not simply an attempt to illuminate the complications of the discourse on borderline disorder for its own sake, but is also animated by the desire to find an answer to these questions: Who is the borderline woman? What is borderline disorder? As I learned more (and learned that this question cannot be answered), my analysis was fueled by a conviction that if the concept lacked a positive referential or even descriptive meaning, other social currents and frameworks must be shaping and constituting its use for certain women patients.

I discuss three phases of meaning of the borderline concept: 1) the late nineteenth century and early medical psychiatry's concept of the "borderland," a term coined by physician Andrew Wynter to designate patients who appeared neither mad nor sane, and yet who were described as socially marginal and transgressing the boundaries of Victorian social codes; 2) post-Freudian psychoanalysis in the United States from 1930 through the 1970s, when the term acquired its meaning within a medical and socially conformist U.S. psychoanalysis, which influenced the shift in focus toward the conscious self-as-object that borderline patients are said to lack; 3) biopsychiatry after 1980, when the category entered the Diagnostic and Statistical Manual of Mental Disorders, the official listing of nomenclature for clinical practice and theory.

The Borderline as Metaphor: Colonizing the "Undefined Wilderness"

The ambiguity of the meaning of the term "borderline" is inherent in the word itself. The term refers to a gap in the logic of psychiatry, rather than a firmly defined essence or identity. As Thomas Aronson writes, "It reflects a weakness in the descriptive language of psychiatry, which often tends to reify its terms, as if they refer to clear, distinct, discrete entities" (Aronson 1985, 219). In its first appearances in the psychoanalytic literature, the borderline category referred to patients who could not be located firmly in any category, and who were said to exhibit a mix of both neurotic and psychotic tendencies, or to vacillate between these states. In current nomenclature, the major defining characteristic of the borderline is instability. Thus, as Louis Sass points out, the diagnosis of any given patient as "borderline" is ambiguous: "Their most central feature, after all, is inconsistency. By definition this means there will not be an obvious and ever-present characteristic by which they can be easily identified" (Sass 1982, 67).

As this statement illustrates, the instability in question refers not only to a given patient's personality or behavior, but to the conceptual status of the borderline construct itself. This dual instability—of the patient's behavior, and of the meaning of the term "borderline"—is expressed in Janice Cauwels's statement that the borderline disorder "not only *causes* instability but also *symbolizes* it" (Cauwels 1992, 82). She titled her book *Imbroglio* in order to symbolize the difficulty and conflict not only of the personality of individuals diagnosed as borderline, but of the debated and controversial status of the term in psychiatry. "Imbroglio," Cauwels points out, can mean a "confused mess," "an acutely painful or embarrassing misunderstanding," or "a violently confused or bitterly complicated altercation." For Cauwels, the image of an imbroglio can represent the difficulty and chaos of the literature on borderline disorder itself. That literature was, by 1992, "voluminous," with four thousand books and articles as of the publication of her book. Cauwels quotes John G. Gunderson, a specialist in borderline disorders, who writes, "The exponential rise in research and the literature defies any one expert's ability to comprehend or master" (Gunderson, in Cauwels 1992, 5). There appear to be as many meanings of the term, Cauwels writes, as there are branches of psychiatry, be they phenomenological, biological, or psychoanalytic. Thomas Aronson argues that "because of the ambiguities and inconsistencies inherent in the multiple meanings of the term, 'borderline' in clinical discourse is commonly used as a label of denigration and obfuscation" (Aronson 1985, 210).

In spite of this instability and inconsistency, many advocates of the use of the term "borderline," while acknowledging the controversy, tend to view the history of the borderline construct as a process of gradual demystification of a real, underlying pathology. Hence, these historians of the borderline construct reproduce what Bryan Turner, following Foucault, calls the "official history of insanity," which is conceptualized as "a series of improvements in knowledge whereby a scientific analysis of insanity eventually emerged as the long-term consequence of the evolution of specific concepts of insanity" (Turner 1987, 60). The change in meanings undergone by the term is attributed to the steady growth of knowledge about the mysteries of the condition itself. This depiction of the scientific exploration of this condition relies on the construction of the borderline as an unexplored territory located between sanity and madness, a realm of the unknown. This is vividly illustrated in a historical overview of the term by Martin Leichtman (1989), who characterizes the image of the borderline disorders as a vast uncharted "territory" of madness that scientific rationality discovered, explored, and demystified by bringing to it the light of scientific reason. Describing the evolution of the concept between the late nineteenth century and 1950, Leichtman writes:

> During those years what have been called borderline disorders
> can be viewed as an uncharted region lying between those
> profound and unmistakable forms of madness that set some
> individuals utterly apart from the rest of humanity and those
> milder forms of psychological disturbance that, however
> peculiar their manifestations, occur in individuals who are
> capable of going about most tasks of day-to-day life and who are
> treatable through some form of outpatient therapy. Those who
> dealt with the borderline concept in this period resemble
> explorers, trappers, and pioneers who ventured out from more
> settled areas to map and cultivate an undefined wilderness.
> (Leichtman 230)

Leichtman's image here is the borderland—the no-man's-land between categories—uncharted and unclaimed territory, waiting to be claimed by scientific discoverers. Yet the explorers—psychiatrists venturing into the unknown—battled with each other over this territory. "To grapple with the borderline concept is to wander onto a battlefield littered with the remains of earlier definitions, fought over by bitterly contending factions, and shelled by other factions who would obliterate the concept altogether in the conviction that it is the devil's handi-work, or, at the least, a holdover from pagan times" (229).

Yet two decades later, writes Leichtman, the wilderness was no longer a wilderness; "it was settled by increasing numbers of clinicians of predominantly psychoanalytic extraction" (232). Later still, with the entrance of the borderline concept into the DSM-III in 1980, "new im-migrants" entered the borderline domain, and "the population of clini-cians and researchers in the borderland grew rapidly. Yet with the rise in population density came numerous complications." The "new im-migrants" were the more medically oriented empirical psychiatrists, who "advanced empirical-descriptive and biological approaches to border-line phenomena and introduced a host of alternative ways to label and conceptualize these conditions" (235).

Here, the borderland metaphor upholds an understanding of this ambiguous category as a real and definable, if vast, territory of mental disturbance. If there is controversy or inconsistency in understanding the borderline disorder, Leichtman's narrative implies, the mysteries of the "wilderness" explain it—not the struggle over meaning arising from competing psychiatric discourses, or even the inherent ambiguity of the word "borderline" itself.

While Leichtman exemplifies a perspective that attributes the shift-ing boundaries of the category of borderline disorders to the unknowns of the condition, these changes can be attributed equally to changes in the organization of psychiatric discourse itself, changes in the types of patients seen, and in the prevailing ideology of mental illness that un-derlies the dominant theories used to explain its causes and manifesta-tions. Definitions of mental disorder change over time, and thus, a particular term will have different referents depending on its particular use. The term "hysteria" for example, has been used to refer to a wide array of symptoms and syndromes over the centuries of its use, from the convulsions believed to be caused by "wandering wombs" by the early Greek physicians, to the paralysis of limbs and other physical, psycho-somatic complaints that Freud and Breuer diagnosed as neurotic, to the description of "hysterical character" in more recent psychoanalytic theory (Satow 1980). These changes can be attributed both to the par-ticular symptoms that are included within a particular category, and to changes in the theories advanced to explain such symptoms.

Thus, concepts of mental illness have a history that it is crucial to examine in order to understand the social construction of psychiatric meaning. The following discussion examines that history in order to trace the shifting ways the concept of "borderline" has been used.

Nineteenth-Century Psychiatry and the Metaphor of the Borderland

The border between sanity and madness, as Foucault shows in *Madness and Civilization*, was historically constructed in the eighteenth century with the emergence of the conception of reason in the classical age in the middle of the seventeenth century. The act that gave rise to the Western conception of "reason" was the "Great Confinement," the removal of those deemed "mad" within asylums, which created a new category of those suffering from "unreason"—the insane. Thus, the conception of reason was dependent on the creation of madness, a madness conceived in the language of reason. The dialogue that medieval and Renaissance culture had carried on with madness was broken off in the creation of the rigid distinction between reason and unreason, and the incarceration of the mad in the specialized setting of the asylum (Foucault 1965).

In the early nineteenth century, this rigid distinction between reason and madness was blurred, as physicians began to recognize some patients who retained their powers of reason, yet nonetheless appeared highly disturbed or showed emotional anguish. They suffered from what Philippe Pinel termed *mania sans delière*, or "moral insanity," defined in 1835 by James Cowles Prichard in England as "madness consisting in a morbid perversion of the natural feelings, affections, inclinations, temper, habits, moral disposition, and natural impulses, without any remarkable disorder or defect of the intellect or knowing and reasoning faculties, and particularly without any insane illusion or hallucination" (Mack 1975). As this broad list reveals, the signs of moral insanity include social deviance. The inclusion of habits and moral disposition reflected the assumptions of Victorian psychiatry, that a lack of will or self-restraint could lead to mental derangement. People displaying a lack of self-control were at risk of insanity.

In defining immorality as mental derangement, early psychiatrists used the metaphor of the borderland. The borderland was a shadowy and ambiguous territory between sanity and madness, where dwelt, as physician Henry Maudsley wrote in 1847, "many persons who, without being insane, exhibit peculiarities of thought, feeling, and character which render them unlike ordinary beings and make them objects of remark among their fellows" (Maudsley 1847, in Showalter 1985, 105). Irving Rosse described the borderland in 1890 as a "class of persons standing in the twilight of right reason and despair—a vast army whose units, consisting of individuals with minds trembling in the balance between reason and madness" (Rosse 1986, 32). Such peculiarities, it was thought, could be expressed by a lack of control of one's "lower nature," and Maudsley, like other physicians, placed emphasis on the lower urban classes and their lack of control as signs of both hereditary regression and of potential lunacy, writing, "There is most madness where there are the fewest ideas, the simplest feelings, and the coarsest desires and ways" (Showalter 1985, 109).

Andrew Wynter, a British physician, depicted the inhabitants of the borderland as able to mask their potential madness. These "incipient lunatics" may "pass about the world with a clean bill of health," yet a trained psychiatrist would be able to spot the signs of hereditary taint that betrayed their evolutionary and moral degeneracy (Showalter 1985, 105). Within this ambiguous and broadly defined realm, those who transgressed nineteenth-century social codes could be spotted as inhabitants of the borderland and at risk of madness. Physicians trained in the language of Darwinist psychiatry looked for the outward physical signs of hereditary taint of madness.

Thus, as John Mack points out, psychiatry was able to annex new realms of behavior as targets of social control. "The concept of moral insanity enabled European and American psychiatrists to consider a vast group of patients and disorders that they had not previously considered as falling within their purview" (Mack 1975, 3). Showalter points out that the metaphor of the borderland reflected the hereditary frameworks of the nineteenth century that legitimated sexual, racial, and class inequalities; those at the "lower rungs" of society were of a lower evolutionary stock. This Darwinian logic was a response to the changing moral atmosphere of the nineteenth century. The borderland, suggests Showalter, "reflected the anxieties of late Victorian psychiatrists, who felt that they were in a temporal and sexual limbo where the traditional boundaries of gender, labor, and behavior were being challenged by New Women and decadent men" (Showalter 1985, 106). Thus, women who defied their feminine "nature" and behaved in ways that transgressed the narrow definitions of women's role—as wife and mother—were at risk of madness. Seeking higher education, in the Darwinian evolutionary framework, drained women's limited energy away from their wombs, leading to nervous prostration and eventual mental derangement.

This annexation of social deviance as mental illness continued into the early twentieth century. In her book *The Psychiatric Persuasion* (1994), which traces the history of the Boston Psychopathic Hospital, Elizabeth Lunbeck describes the new category of "psychopathy" to encompass a wide range of antisocial behavior as a legitimate focus of psychiatry: "Psychiatrists entered the public sphere aggressively promoting an agenda of defect and difference that they provocatively cast as a wholesale assault on the egalitarian heritage of the Enlightenment. Proposing to identify defect where others saw soundness, difference where ideologues saw sameness, psychiatrists staked their claim to the uncharted territory that they argued lay between frank manifestations of disease on the one hand and indisputable normality on the other" (62).

Psychopathy, or psychopathic personality, was the newly invented category. "Psychopathy at its simplest rendered a range of behaviors beyond the mental tests' measure—eccentricities, peculiarities, oddities, quirks—as sign of innate defect and brought them within the psychiatrist's purview. Psychopathy was . . . usefully but dangerously indeterminate, a rubric that comfortably encompassed incarcerated criminals and dissipated high-livers, promiscuous girls and lazy men, deficiencies so various, so numerous, and, in the end, so elusive that some wondered whether it referred to anything at all" (65). Lunbeck points out that the only certainty about this category was its general meaning as "abnormality": "In the end, psychiatrists could only specify what psychopathy was—and they were sure it was something—by reference to what it was not, and that was normality" (68).

The term "psychopathy" became more narrowly defined between 1910 and 1930, referring only to antisocial behaviors, eclipsing the more diffuse conditions not having to do with antisocial qualities. These other, more broadly defined conditions were neglected as a focus until the 1930s, when psychoanalysts become interested in the patients who showed particularly severe forms of disturbance. The subsequent development of the concept of the borderline occurred primarily within psychoanalysis, as it developed in the United States starting in the 1930s.

Beyond Oedipus: The Borderline in Psychoanalysis

A second phase in the development of the borderline concept occurred within psychoanalysis in North America, where analysts began seeing patients who, as Adolph Stern wrote, "fit frankly neither into the psychotic nor into the psychoneurotic group" (Stern 1938, 467). Stern noted that the number of such patients was increasing, and that analytic treatment methods were unsuccessful with this group.

In this period, analysts tended to describe such patients only by reference to other, adjacent categories, such as schizophrenia. Later, as the discourse on the borderline case grew, more systematic attempts to map out the characteristics and underlying dynamics of the borderline character appeared. Rather than depicting it as either a severe neurosis or a weak or pseudo form of schizophrenia, it was framed as a unique entity in its own right, a distinctive character type.

The early European Freudians had confronted certain patients who were difficult or whose disturbance appeared to go beyond typical neurosis. Wilhelm Reich, for example, had treated patients who resisted the aims of analytic investigation of unconscious memories. Reich viewed this resistance as an "armor" of "character" that had to be confronted and interpreted in order to proceed with the analysis. Reich, like Freud and other analysts, among them Franz Alexander, had developed a typology of discrete character types linked to the ego and its defenses, including the impulsive, hysterical, masochistic, and neurotic character types. Reich wrote that the impulsive and neurotic character "constitute borderline cases between psychosis and health" (Mack 1975, 6).

While Freud and other European Freudians had begun to conceptualize character types, the concept of borderline (and narcissistic) character types occurred primarily in the United States. Historians of the borderline case attribute this to the close relationship between psychoanalysis and medical psychiatry in the United States since its introduction in the early part of the twentieth century. Psychoanalysts became an elite part of the American Psychiatric Association by the 1930s, just twenty years after Freud's first visit to the United States in 1909, when he delivered a series of lectures at Clark University in Worcester, Massachusetts. Psychoanalytic concepts were widely embraced in U.S. departments of psychiatry, and influential physicians such as Adolf Meyer, James Jackson Putnam, G. Stanley Hall, William Alanson White, and others introduced Freudian concepts into their own psychiatric hospital treatment (Stone 1986). Psychoanalytically trained psychiatrists saw a range of patient types within hospitals, and applied Freudian concepts not only to milder cases but to the more severe cases as well. Hence there was an interest in delineating the borderline cases along the spectrum of neurosis and psychosis.

In the 1930s and 1940s, when European analysts fleeing Nazism entered U.S. departments of psychiatry, analytic thinking on the borderline case developed further. Émigré analysts, such as Adolph Stern, Helene Deutsch, and Gregory Zilboorg, recognized a large group of patients in their clinical practices that were not overtly psychotic, but who nonetheless suffered major difficulties in self-esteem and who showed high levels of anxiety and depression. While they did not always use the label "borderline" (with the exception of Stern), these analysts concentrated on the psychic conflicts underlying this large group of patients. Analysts confronting such patients proposed new theories of psychic development that went beyond Freud's psychosexual stage theory, either replacing it with new propositions or accommodating its insights to the conceptual framework of Freudian theory (Greenberg and Mitchell 1983).

The first detailed description of the borderline case is found in Adolph Stern's 1938 paper, which he read for the New York Psychoanalytic Society. He describes a type of analysand who deviates significantly from the classic neurotic patients that has typified analytic treatment. "It is well known," he writes, "that a large group of patients fit frankly neither into the psychotic nor into the psychoneurotic group, and that this border line group of patients is extremely difficult to handle effectively by any psychotherapeutic method" (Stern 1938, 467). In contrast to the neurotic patient, the borderline's anxiety has its source not in psychosexual impulses, but in narcissism: "an investigation of the earliest narcissistic periods in very early childhood discloses factors adversely affecting their narcissistic development. . . . Because of [these] experiences this group never develops a sense of security acquired by being loved, which is the birthright of every child. These patients suffer from affective (narcissistic) malnutrition" (470). Following Freud's terminology, Stern refers to these cases as "narcissistic neuroses." Many of the borderline patients have had childhoods characterized by family quarreling, divorce, or worse: "Actual cruelty, neglect and brutality by the parents of many years' duration are factors found in these patients. These factors operate more or less constantly over many years from earliest childhood. They are not single experiences" (470). The borderline group suffers from insecurity and anxiety, feelings of inferiority, hypersensitivity, and negative reactions to the therapy.

Stern does not discuss differences between women and men, and makes brief mention only of the conventional Freudian understanding of the roots of disturbance, the Oedipus Complex: "These adults in their childhood as a rule were inordinately submissive and obedient through fear and need. They clung to parents and substitutes with the desperation of the greatly endangered. In the female, penis envy and in the male, castration anxiety play considerable roles. Anxiety because of the sexual impulse also plays a considerable role. The Oedipus complex most assuredly does" (477). However, Stern goes on to note that in contrast to the neurotic patient, the borderline patients suffer from a higher degree of oedipal insecurity.

Other analysts focused on patients in analysis who appeared more disturbed than classic neurotics. Many of these early post-Freudian analysts understood these cases as modified forms of schizophrenia, and their language reflects it. Gregory Zilboorg, for example, felt that cases that were considered borderline were in fact cases of schizophrenia masked by an outwardly normal appearance, and that it would not be difficult "to discern a schizophrenia under whatever guise we choose to consider a pathological phenomena to appear: a compulsion neurosis, a borderline case, an 'incipient' schizophrenia, or even a hysteria" (Zilboorg 1941, 151). Zilboorg's view of such patients echoes the nineteenth-century physicians' depiction of those who inhabited the borderland as "incipient lunatics," able, as Andrew Wynter notes, to "pass about the world with a clean bill of health" (Showalter 1985, 105). "Stated briefly, the psychological picture of a schizophrenia may not present any striking appearance at all. The individual may appear normal in all respects, even suave and almost worldly; he may sometimes give the impression of a warm personality" (Zilboorg 1941, 152).

And yet this outward normality belies a world of inner turmoil. These patients are "suffused with hatred" and are constantly aware of "physical tension" and anxiety. Such individuals, Zilboorg concluded, "remain more or less on the loose in the actual or figurative sense, outwardly and inwardly; hence the suggested designation of ambulatory schizophrenias" (152).

The "difficult" patient in analysis was unpredictable and often uncooperative. This example from analyst Melitta Schmideberg is illustrative:

> The majority of my patients suffer neither from a classical neurosis nor a definite psychosis. They are "difficult" and may or may not have circumscribed neurotic symptoms. Most of them would probably be diagnosed as "psychopaths" or "borderline cases." . . . Such patients are unable to stand routine and regularity. They transgress every rule; naturally they do not attend treatment regularly, are late for their appointments and, when they do appear, are unreliable about payments. They do not associate freely and often do not talk at all. They refuse to lie on the couch. They often come for analysis only under persuasion or pressure and even when they come on their own, their insight does not last nor carry them through difficulties. . . . It is difficult to establish emotional contact or, alternately, the transference is most unreliable. The patient may appear deeply attached one day and not turn up the next. The speed with which his mood changes from one extreme to another is uncanny. In one case, it was literally a question of seconds. (Schmideberg 1947, in Stone 1986, 92)

During the 1950s, the usefulness of the conception was hotly debated. Many analysts objected to the diagnosis. During an all-day panel in May 1954 devoted to the borderline case, Gregory Zilboorg questioned whether the borderline state existed at all: "We seem to seek we know not yet quite clearly what" (Rangell 1955, 285). On the same panel, Elizabeth Zetzel objected to the borderline concept, on the grounds that there is no sharp line of differentiation between neurosis and psychosis, and that the term "border area" might be more accurate. She also stated that the term "borderline" tended to be used as a "wastebasket" term that prevented finer or more subtle diagnostic states (Rangell 1955, 289).

Yet the concept had its supporters. Jan Frank argued that there was indeed a borderline state and that it was manifest in the widespread increase in "delinquency, road killings, and what appears to be the schizophrenization of mankind," which he described as an inability to neutralize aggressive or sexual energy that is directed outward. Frank regretted the passage of the Victorian era and the syndrome of hysteria. "That woman were prone to swoon at that time was better than the prevalence of borderline cases today. The latter can be attributed largely as an etiologic factor to the dissolution of the family as a unit, which was brought about in part by two World Wars and which cannot be replaced by mental hygiene" (Rangell 1955, 290).

The Borderline as Unstable Self

The meaning of the borderline category is crystallized during the 1950s and 1960s, with the term taking on a specialized clinical meaning as a distinct character, ego, or personality type, rather than merely designating a descriptive location between categories.

While the earlier cases emphasized social maladjustment broadly conceived, in the 1950s the theme of ego instability and fragmentation of self began to be emphasized. During this decade, discussions of the connection of the borderline condition to schizophrenia began to wane, as the largely descriptive accounts of the borderline case in the 1940s gave way to the more detailed discussions of the underlying psychic conflicts and dynamics of the borderline condition. The focus on ego adjustment reflected the wider trend in popularity of the "ego psychology" school of psychoanalysis, advocated by Freud's daughter Anna Freud. Ego psychology shifted emphasis away from the study of the unconscious and toward the study of the ego's overall functioning and its mechanisms of coping and adapting to the outside world.

In 1953, Robert P. Knight published what Michael Stone (1986) refers to as a "watershed" article on the borderline condition, which focuses not on its possible masking of schizophrenia, but on the specific ego weaknesses of the borderline patient. Knight states that the borderline patient's ego functioning, which he describes as "secondary process thinking, integration, realistic planning adaptation to the environment, maintenance of object relationships, and defenses against primitive unconscious impulses" is "severely weakened" (Knight, in Stone 1986, 165). Knight likens the ego to a defensive army, which in borderline patients is "retreating," while various defensive symptoms represent a sort of advance guard, protecting the fragile and retreating ego: "Various segments or detachments of the retreating army may make a stand and conduct holding or delaying operations at various points where the terrain lends itself to such operations, while the main retreating forces may have retired much farther to the rear. . . . The superficial clinical picture—hysteria, phobia, obsessions, compulsive rituals—may represent a holding operation in a forward position, while the major portion of the ego has regressed far behind this in varying degrees of disorder" (164).

The 1960s saw further development of the borderline category as a discrete entity in its own right, rather than as a disguised form of schizophrenia. The major focus of the psychoanalytic literature during this period, drawing on Knight's earlier work, was a description of the borderline patient as lacking a stable self. The evolution of the concept from that designating its border with other categories to its status as a discrete entity, a discernible "ego" or "personality" organization, culminates in Otto Kernberg's approach to the borderline conditions. Kernberg's achievement, writes Stone,

> was to assemble the various conceptual fragments provided by his predecessors into a coherent picture, clinically more useful and diagnostically more precise than the at times colorful but all too often amorphous descriptions of the past. The trend toward the establishment of borderline disorders as constituting a separate and discriminable entity also finds its most coherent expression in Kernberg's writing: borderline personality organization, as he was to call it, is now equipped with inclusion criteria and exclusion criteria. (Stone 1986, 152)

Kernberg's assemblage of the "conceptual fragments" of the borderline construct solidified the two trends that can be discerned in Knight's work: First was the construction of the borderline condition as a defensive ego or personality type—a recognizable "borderline personality organization." Second, Kernberg provided a fuller theory of the roots of the disorder in early childhood, and more specifically in early infancy—the pre-oedipal period. This early period was the source of the borderline patient's unstable self.

In Kernberg's account, the major difference between the neurotic patient and the borderline patient is the borderline's lack of a clear sense of identity. Unlike the neurotic patient, who is able to provide a verbal portrait of self, borderline patients are not able to provide a coherent description of themselves. Their descriptions, Kernberg states, are contradictory, vague, or incomplete. In addition, their behavior is inconsistent. One major symptom is "splitting," in which one holds two contradictory perceptions of the self or others as either all good or all bad, and is unable to integrate them into a coherent total image. The patient is said to vacillate from one image to the other. Splitting is said to originate in the patient's early unconscious responses to the mother, when the child's perception of her as nurturing and gratifying are kept separate from perceptions of her as depriving or punitive. This initial defense against contradictory images of the mother later becomes a defense mechanism in the patient's relations with others.

For Kernberg, evidence that a patient is using this splitting mechanism appears in the patient's reaction toward the analyst. One of Kernberg's patients, a woman in her thirties, reacted to Kernberg in an inconsistent fashion, as he describes in an interview: "In one session, the patient may experience me as the most helpful, loving, understanding human being and may feel totally relieved and happy, and all the problems are solved. Three sessions later, she may berate me as the most ruthless, indifferent, manipulative person she has ever met. Total unhappiness about the treatment, ready to drop it and never come back" (Kernberg, quoted in Sass 1982, 66).

Borderline personality organization is characterized by what Kernberg calls "immature" ego defense-mechanisms, which include not only "splitting" but also "magical thinking" or the use of superstitions, phobias, and obsessive-compulsive behavior; feelings of omnipotence; projection of one's unpleasant characteristics onto others, and finally "projective identification," in which the person perceives and identifies with the projected characteristics.

While Kernberg's writing exemplifies the trend toward conceptualizing the borderline as a discrete entity, this "ego organization" was still positioned between neurosis and psychosis. Kernberg posited a hierarchy of personality, from normality through neurosis to psychosis, with borderline personality occupying the middle level between neurosis and psychosis. As Thomas Aronson states, Kernberg is most representative of the current psychoanalytic conception of the borderline as a "level of function or ego organization between neurosis and psychosis. . . . Psychostructurally, borderline patients exist in the borderland between neurosis and psychosis. In other words, modern analytic authors . . . see it as in a distinct class by itself, while at the same time on a continuum with neurotic and psychotic functioning. It is neither a mild form of a major psychiatric disorder nor a personality disorder, but rather a stable middle level of ego organization separate from neurosis and psychosis" (Aronson 1985, 216). For individuals diagnosed as borderline, their borderland position is located within, as a pathological ego structure.

This borderland pathological ego structure, moreover, is rooted in the person's earliest childhood. Kernberg's theory of the childhood roots of the borderline condition is part of a major shift in emphasis in post-Freudian psychoanalysis: the growing influence of object relations theory, which focuses on the earliest stages of life when a fundamental sense of self is formed, and an awareness of the distinction between the self and the external world. The origins of borderline disorder (as well as the closely related disorder, narcissistic personality disorder) are said to lie in this early period of self/other recognition.

In its focus on early childhood, object relations theory gives the mother a pivotal role in determining the shape of the infant's personality. The fragile process of relating to and differentiating from the mother in the pre-oedipal period is the primary site for the construction of a sense of self or identity. Thus, any aberrations in "good enough" mothering will prove disastrous for the fragile emerging self. It is not surprising, then, that "inadequate mothering" or "maternal deprivation" have been widely accepted as the main causes of the "disorders of the self." Symptoms of borderline or narcissistic conditions are said to embody this failed relationship.

While borderline disorder was beginning to be defined as ego weakness or identity fragmentation during the 1960s, it continued to be associated with social marginality, and psychiatrists continued to place certain patients in this uncertain borderland. In a 1966 paper, "The Psychotherapy of Borderland Patients," Richard Chessick notes that these patients "seem to lie on the periphery of psychiatry, on the periphery of society, and on the periphery of penology. Some of them have been in and out of prisons as well as mental hospitals and have had repeated brushes with the police for various reasons" (Chessick 1966, 600). Chessick notes that there were two groups of patients: First were the "borderline" or "pan-neurotic" cases, all but one of whom were women; and the second group consisted of patients with addictions of various sorts (drug, alcohol, or food). All but two in the addictions group were males. Chessick writes, "Many of them had previously received various forms of treatment with no noticeable results. Others were referred as 'addicts' with the implication that they were untreatable because of their condition. There were four 'alcoholics' and two patients diagnosed as 'chronic schizophrenics' who were referred with the advice that they be permanently put in the state hospital" (600).

In spite of Kernberg's synthesis of literature on the borderline, a diversity of approaches continued to proliferate. By the late 1970s, serious discrepancies appeared in the different psychoanalytic and psychiatric models of the borderline personality. One study reviewed four sets of criteria for borderline disorder and found a total of 104 different criteria identified for borderline disorder, encompassing the patient's mental status, history, interpersonal relationships, and defense mechanisms. Of these, only one—referring to the patient's behavior in the interview as appearing "adaptive and appropriate"—was agreed on by the four authors. Further, half of the 104 criteria were present in only one of the four authors' sets of diagnostic criteria. The authors conclude, "For 'the borderline patient' concept, the multiplicity of diagnostic terms suggests the question whether these terms are referring to the same clinical population or not . . . In one way or another, it seems as if the whole range of psychopathology of personality is represented" (Perry and Klerman 1978, 150).

Another study that reviewed patient charts found that of twenty charts reviewed, nine different borderline diagnoses were used, including borderline, borderline state, borderline personality, borderline syndrome, borderline psychosis, borderline schizophrenia, borderline schizoid personality, borderline hysterical character, and borderline character (Rich 1978).

Thus, while Kernberg and others were working on systematizing the borderline category by defining it as a distinct personality type, the word "borderline" continued to be applied in diverse ways. It remained for the developers of the new edition of the Diagnostic and Statistical Manual of Mental Disorders, the DSM-III, to further codify the diagnosis. With its redefinition in the DSM-III as a personality disorder, the focus on underlying character or self was codified in the official nomenclature.

The Borderline Personality Disorder in Psychiatry

During the 1970s, at the same time that Kernberg and others were developing theories of the borderline personality, work was under way to develop a new, revised edition of the Diagnostic and Statistical Manual of Mental Disorders. The third edition of the DSM was published in 1980 by the American Psychiatric Association (APA 1980). The DSM defines the codes that are used for insurance reimbursement of mental health care, and is thus used in a wide range of mental health and health care settings. It was in this third edition that the borderline category first appeared as "borderline personality disorder."

The entry of the borderline diagnosis in the DSM in 1980 marked a watershed in its conceptual history. For the first time, the borderline diagnosis was included in the official psychiatric nomenclature, thereby gaining wide legitimacy and greater visibility within the mental health field as a discrete psychiatric category. Further, the definition appearing in the 1980 version of the DSM marked a shift away from psychoanalytic formulations of the concept toward a largely empirical medical definition. Rather than emphasizing underlying psychodynamic processes, the new medical definition focused on observable behaviors (Aronson 1985). The developers of the DSM-III based the criteria for borderline personality disorder on a large study of over eight hundred patients diagnosed as borderline. Based on factor analysis of the symptoms of these patients, the main criterion for the diagnosis as it appeared in the DSM-III was identified: instability "in sense of identity, interpersonal relationships, impulse control, and mood and affect regulation" (Spitzer, Williams, and Skodol 1980, 162).

This empirical focus is consistent with what Philip Brown (1990) terms the "neo-Kraepelinian" aims of contemporary diagnosis, modeled on Emil Kraepelin's nineteenth-century attempt to develop a complete taxonomy of mental disorders. Thus, the borderline diagnosis takes on a new behavioral meaning.

The visibility of borderline personality disorder was further heightened by the mandate contained in this new psychiatric classification to record personality disorders on a separate diagnostic dimension for all patients, regardless of their primary diagnosis. The personality disorders were to be recorded on a separate diagnostic axis or dimension, known as Axis II. The effect of this emphasis on personality in psychiatric diagnosis was to medicalize it, creating new terrain for psychiatric scrutiny and treatment.

Together, these two changes to the DSM had the effect of raising awareness about borderline personality disorder and of increasing the rates of the diagnosis. By 1984, four years after the publication of DSM-III, borderline personality disorder was the most commonly diagnosed personality disorder (Gunderson and Zanarini 1987, 8).

To explain the rapid rise of the visibility of borderline personality disorders within psychiatric discourse, the new prominence given to personality within the DSM must be examined.

THE PERSONALITY AS PATHOLOGY

The boundaries between particular disorders, far from being static reflections of some objectively existing and observable behavior, are always being contested, defined, and redefined in light of new theories. In this view, the definition of mental disorder, like the construction of any social problem, is a political process, with the various disciplines of medical psychiatry, psychoanalysis, psychology, and social work participating in an ongoing debate over terms.

As an explicit standardization of the heterogeneous meanings that notions of mental disorder take on in various guises, the DSM has a large hand in shaping the way clinicians in diverse professions perceive troubled individuals. Joel Kovel, in a critique of the epistemological consequences of the DSM-III, points out that implicit in the DSM-III is the structure of the impersonal and expert gaze that makes invisible the impact of the psychiatric institution itself in creating its object of investigation (Kovel 1988).

The development of the DSM-III is a prime example of the conflicts and turf wars that underlay the contemporary attempt to define and order mental disorders. Theodore Millon, a psychologist and member of the APA Task Force charged with developing the categories for the DSM-III, provides a telling background to the conflicts that occurred in the five-year development of the DSM's third edition (Millon 1983). These include conflicts between psychiatrists and psychologists over a planned medical definition of mental disorder, and the controversial decision to remove the psychoanalytic term "neurosis" from the manual altogether. Within this contested terrain of conflicting definitions and semantic challenge, the definition of disorders themselves takes place, as diagnostic criteria, the rules of definition on what is to be included and what excluded in a particular disorder, are developed. New categories are created, existing categories are further split into finer classes, and some categories (such as homosexuality, voted out of the DSM-III in 1980) are removed.

Ironically, it was the challenge by psychologists to the dominant medical or disease model of mental illness that led its constructors to add the personality onto the diagnostic system. This provided new terrain for medicalization of the person—the now distinct "personality." The major change that shifted DSM-III away from a disease model was its inclusion of several contextual, longitudinal elements in the diagnostic schema, the personality being the most important of these. This is what is known as the multiaxial format, one that Millon states is no less than a paradigm shift in diagnosis, representing a "distinct turn from the traditional medical disease model where the clinician's job is to

disentangle and clear away 'distracting' symptoms and signs so as to pin-
point the underlying or 'true' pathophysiologic state" (Miller 1983, 809).
A person is diagnosed not on one dimension (that is, the main clinical
problem that is the ostensible cause for admission or consultation) but
on five dimensions: the main mental disorder traditionally conceived
(Axis I), plus four additional axes or dimensions: the personality traits
or disorders (Axis II); any relevant physical condition (Axis III); "psychosocial stressors" (Axis IV), and finally, the person's "highest level
of adaptive functioning in the past year" (Axis V). Axis IV and Axis
V, however, were made optional.

For Millon, these additional dimensions of information about a patient are highly significant in that they orient the observer toward the
person instead of the "disease entity." The inclusion of these elements,
he writes, directs the clinician to address "an entire panorama of contextual dimensions, notably the person's overall style of psychological
functioning [the personality], the qualities of a person's current situational environment, and his or her strengths and potentials for con-
structive and healthy coping" (810). Millon stresses "context" in his
assessment of the multiple dimensions: these elements provide a context within which the disorder, often more transient, unfolds and is sus-
tained; hence, information about that context helps the observing
clinician understand the disorder in a fuller sense.

The personality is one such contextual element (Axis II), defined
by Millon as the "enduring and often more prosaic styles of personality
functioning" (810). The DSM-III's definition of personality disorder is
in accord with the general definition of mental disorder: "either significant impairment in social or occupational functioning or subjective
distress" (APA 1980, 305). It is important to note that of the three contextual axes, only Axis II, the personality disorder, is a required element. The personality disorders, though existing in prior DSMs (for
example, the diagnoses paranoid personality, obsessive-compulsive, antisocial, and passive-aggressive personality existed in the DSM-II) are
now separated out, and clinicians are encouraged to record a personality disorder for all patients. Millon points out that the task force encouraged the formal notation of all relevant personality traits on Axis
II, "even when a distinctive personality 'disorder' was not in evidence"
(810). Hence, this dimension of personality is now a significant fea-

ture of the way mental health professionals perceive and treat their clients.

BORDERLINE PERSONALITY DISORDER: THE OFFICIAL DEFINITION
Borderline personality disorder was one of six new personality disorders included in the new edition: avoidant, dependent, narcissistic, schizoid, borderline, and schizotypal personalities. An existing category, predominantly applied to women, termed "hysterical personality disorder," was changed to "histrionic personality disorder."

The final definition of the disorder is a checklist of eight symptoms, including emotional instability, inappropriate or intense anger, self-destructive acts; impulsivity, unstable relationships, identity disturbance, and chronic feelings of emptiness or boredom (APA 1980, 346). Janice Cauwels points out that the DSM-III definition has been criticized as being too broad: "As Dr. Stone points out, the definition allows for 93 possible combinations of criteria . . . so that some DSM-III-R borderlines hardly resemble others" (Cauwels 1992, 66).

The mandate contained in the DSM-III to record personality traits for all patients, and the creation of a new category for borderline personality, had the effect of propelling the disorder into visibility and generated widespread interest in the disorder. The creators of the DSM-III cited as a major achievement the creation of reliable and uniform diagnostic criteria (Spitzer, Williams, and Skodol 1980). For new categories of personality disorder, comparable research studies were facilitated for the first time. This was possible because researchers were speaking about the same entity in different settings (the possibilities that these standardized criteria are applied differently notwithstanding). As Millon notes, "the 'borderline' pattern will no longer be characterized one way at Massachusetts General Hospital, another at the Menninger Clinic, a third at Michael Reese Hospital, and a fourth at the Langley Porter Institute" (Millon 1983, 808).

This may account for the large increase in the volume of research articles on personality disorders in the years between 1975 and 1985. The literature on the topic of personality disorders more than tripled in size between 1975 and 1985, from 69 articles in 1975 to 262 articles in 1985. Much of this expanded increase and visibility of writing on personality disorders can be attributed to an expanded interest in the borderline personality. Overall, the number of articles specifically devoted to borderline personality disorder jumped from only 11 in 1975 to 88 in 1985 (Blashfield and McElroy 1987, 544). While antisocial personality had been the focus of the bulk of the 1975 articles, (37 percent of the articles), with borderline the focus of only 18 percent of the articles, by 1985 it was borderline personality disorder that predominated in the literature (40 percent of the articles), with antisocial personality accounting for only 25 percent of research articles.

The effect of separating out a diagnostic axis for the personality traits has the ultimate effect of expanding the terrain of what is to be considered an "illness": the personality, particularly the person's unstable sense of self. While for Millon this new focus on enduring personality traits represents an advance in its turn toward contextual elements, the overall effect may be quite different. The personality structure, inferred to exist from the person's verbal and nonverbal behaviors, is new terrain for medicalization.

Labeling the "Difficult Patient"

Within the proliferating discourse on the borderline diagnosis, debate continues over the meaning of the term, the patients to whom it is applied, and the theoretical explanations offered for the causes of emotional instability and identity conflicts. Despite the DSM developers' attempts to create a consistent meaning for the borderline category, its actual application remains ambiguous. As Dana Becker writes, "It is my impression that although empirical research on borderline personality disorder, using actual patients or case records for the collection of data, employs some rigor in ensuring that those studied fulfill criteria for the borderline diagnosis, many practitioners are looser in their use of borderline as a descriptive term and, probably, looser in their adherence to strict diagnostic accuracy" (Becker 1997, xiv).

Further, the use of the borderline diagnosis as a label of denigration for particularly troublesome patients has remained a concern of both advocates and critics of the term. For example, one study found that nurses showed less empathy or emotional involvement with hypothetical patients diagnosed as borderline than with those diagnosed schizophrenic (Gallop, Lancee, and Garfinkel 1989). Another critical review of the diverse ways the borderline diagnosis is used in clinical practice states that the borderline diagnosis is particularly vulnerable to multiple uses, for several reasons: 1) The criteria for borderline disorder "seem to depend on one's theoretical orientation"; 2) the term is new; only recently has it been deemed a useful and homogeneous category outside the specialized setting of psychoanalysis; and 3) "patients who have a borderline personality structure often have symptoms (e.g., emotional lability, suicidal and/or homicidal ideation or behavior, serious interpersonal problems, and rage) that are difficult to tolerate, let alone treat" (Reiser and Levenson 1984, 1528). As a result, the borderline diagnosis is commonly used as a derogatory label, an expression of "countertransference hate":

> Repeatedly, we have heard therapists in these institutional settings refer to a wide and markedly heterogeneous group of patients as "just a bunch of borderlines." Used this way, the term "borderline" loses all theoretical meaning and simply becomes the latest institutional epithet—another colloquial expression of contempt, like "gomer," "crock," or "turkey." When slang takes the form of pseudo-scientific jargon, however, counter-transference hatred becomes disguised as a technical term, making it doubly dangerous. (1528)

Thus, in spite of claims for a new level of consistency in the DSM-III version of borderline disorder, controversy persists among clinicians as to the meaning of the term, and the ways the term is applied in specific cases.

The Feminization of the Borderline

What remains to be explored is how gender figures into the genealogy of the borderline concept. What is the relationship of gender in the delineation of this new, troubled and unstable patient? And how does borderline instability become associated with femininity and with women?

While in the early years of psychoanalysis, both male and female patients were described, the later descriptions feature predominantly women. In an early paper (1941), Gregory Zilboorg notes that his borderline patients, whom he has described as "ambulatory schizophrenics," are mostly men:

> It will be noted that I have been speaking here of men. I do not know whether as a result of fortuitous circumstances my experience has been limited only to men of this psychological variety, or whether this psychopathological state is met with mostly in men. My observations include extremely few women of this type, and these have shown a greater tendency toward agitated and more vivid depressive trends. One must add that all such cases, men and women but particularly men, are very frequently preoccupied with thoughts of suicide, and they are just as apt to kill someone else as to kill themselves. (Zilboorg 1941, 152)

Yet other analysts in the early period of psychoanalysis focused primarily on female patients. In 1942, in an article that, as Michael Stone writes, "laid the foundation for contemporary psychoanalytic formulations of the borderline" (Stone 1986, 48), Helene Deutsch describes a group of women patients who appear to exhibit a superficiality and inner emptiness in their personalities. Deutsch calls this type of patient the "as if" personality: "My only reason for using so unoriginal a label for the type of person I wish to present is that every attempt to understand the way of feeling and manner of life of this type forces on the observer the inescapable impression that the individual's whole relationship to life has something about it which is lacking in genuineness and yet outwardly runs along 'as if' it were complete. Even the layman sooner or later inquires, after meeting such an 'as if' patient: what is wrong with him, or her?" (Deutsch, in Stone 1986, 75).

Such persons, Deutsch notes, appear to be "normal" yet, on closer observation, lack warmth or depth: "It is like the performance of an actor who is technically well trained but who lacks the necessary spark to make his impersonations true to life" (76).

The "as if" personality shows a "completely passive attitude to the environment with a highly plastic readiness to pick up signals from the outer world and to mold oneself and one's behavior accordingly" (77). In the place of a personality, there is only mimicry of others, and an identification with the environment that facilitates "good adaptation" to the world without depth or inner life. "If it is a woman, she seems to be the quintessence of feminine devotion, an impression which is particularly imparted by her passivity and readiness for identification. Soon, however, the lack of real warmth brings such an emptiness and dullness to the emotional atmosphere that the man as a rule precipitously breaks off the relationship" (77).

Deutsch believes that the "as if" personality may have represented a phase leading up to the onset of schizophrenia, but she states that her patients "do not belong among the commonly accepted forms of neurosis, and they are too well adjusted to reality to be called psychotic" (90).

In 1949, Paul Hoch and Phillip Polatin used a concept of disguised schizophrenia, which they termed "pseudoneurotic schizophrenia," to refer to certain patients who showed a deeper level of anxiety and a wider variety of symptoms than the neurotic (Hoch and Polatin 1949). Like Deutsch's, their patients were predominantly women. They describe patients whose symptoms include "ambivalence," which is "not localized, but it is diffuse and widespread involving the patient's aims, his social adaptation and his sexual adjustment;" "polymorphous anxiety"; and a combination of all the symptoms of neurosis that they term "pan-neurosis" (250).

Within this wide array of symptoms, the theme of social adjustment, particularly in relation to gender positioning, is a prominent one. Hoch and Polatin describe several cases, including a twenty-one-year-old woman suffering from depression and anorexia; and two women who appear to be experiencing gender conflicts: a twenty-nine-year-old woman who experiences "feelings of unreality and depersonalization" that include "the idea that she was becoming more like a man," and another female patient who states, "I have a male mind and a female body and I don't like women" (268). One woman feels she is becoming two persons: "She began to think of herself at times very objectively; and she would smile at her own activities and reactions. She also could hear herself talk to her self as if there were two persons. At times she would laugh at her own feelings" (274).

Gender conflict is a theme that also appears in Chessick's later account of "borderland" patients (Chessick 1966). Writing of the mostly female "pan-neurotic" patients, he describes how it is crucial to uncover patients' "pet and secret narcissistic fantasies":

For example, one patient secretly felt that she was a male in female's clothing. She felt that her outer appearance of femininity was an additional weapon in the dreadful jungle of the world that she had to live in. Thus, by using seduction and sexuality, she could trap unwitting males into becoming slaves and then break them down so that they begged her to stay with them. In effect, what she was doing was reversing the situation of her childhood where her extremely destructive mother kept her in a trapped and helpless situation. The secret fantasy was that she was some kind of superhuman being who did not have the real genitals and figure of a female but who kept this fact hidden underneath female clothing. (Chessick 1966, 603)

By the late 1970s and early 1980s, the majority of cases discussed in the clinical literature were women (Boyer 1977; Chessick 1982; Flax 1986; Ross 1976; Singer 1977b). When borderline personality disorder appeared in the DSM in 1980, the predominance of women was explicitly acknowledged in the definition: "The disorder is more commonly diagnosed in women" (APA 1980, 347).

Sexual Abuse and the Feminization of the Borderline

The issue of feminization is a complex one. At issue are the ways psychiatric discourse organizes and names women's expressed symptoms, and how such labels change over time. It is important to emphasize here that the construct or label has shifted over time in the direction of stereotypically defined feminine traits, and, regardless of whether we can say that more women experience such symptoms, the label captures, names, and codifies such symptoms.

One particular dimension of women's experience that appears to be captured by the current definition is childhood sexual abuse and its effects manifest in later psychological disturbance. Some researchers have found that a high proportion of borderline patients have histories of childhood sexual abuse, neglect, or emotional abuse. One study comparing borderline with other patients found that significantly more borderline patients had histories of trauma, including suffering physical abuse (71 percent) and sexual abuse (68 percent), and witnessing serious domestic violence (62 percent) (Herman, Perry, and van der Kolk

1989, 491). In a review of studies, Cauwels notes that the proportion of borderline patients with childhood sexual abuse histories ranges from 30 to 70 percent (Cauwels 1992, 242). Herman, Perry, and van der Kolk note that since girls are at two to three times greater risk for sexual victimization, sexual abuse is an important element that could explain the higher prevalence of borderline personality disorder in women.

Some observers, noting the high percentage of borderline patients with abuse histories, argue that many of the symptoms associated with borderline personality may be responses to the abuse, and may in fact be better defined as post-traumatic stress disorder (PTSD). The symptoms of PTSD overlap considerably with those of borderline personality disorder, and focus on unstable emotions, behavior, and relationships (Cauwels 1992, 85). Herman posits that the behaviors associated with borderline personality disorder may be one form of adaptation to trauma, with the most prominent aspect being the "disturbance in identity and relationship" (Herman 1992, 126). Borderline is among the most prominent psychiatric diagnoses, along with somatization disorder and multiple personality disorder, given to women suffering from childhood trauma. The symptoms of each of these diagnoses, Herman notes, were at one time subsumed under the obsolete category of hysteria. Given the range of responses to trauma, Herman argues that even the category of PTSD is too narrowly defined, focusing on singular events such as combat, disaster, and rape, thus missing the more complex picture of prolonged abuse. She proposes a new category to encompass the spectrum of conditions related to trauma: "complex post-traumatic stress disorder" (119).

Prominent researchers on the borderline disorder have acknowledged that they have missed the significance of sexual abuse in their borderline patients. Joel Paris states, "I have kicked myself because I have heard sexual abuse histories from my patients for 15 or 20 years but didn't write about it (Cauwels 1992, 243). John Gunderson also noted, "I am among those people . . . whose theorizing failed to give abuse the attention it very clearly deserves" (243).

Judith Herman notes that the most prominent theorist on borderline disorder, Otto Kernberg, minimized the importance of sexual abuse as a source of some of the symptoms of the borderline disorders. "In 1985, Dr. Kernberg headed a discussion group at the annual convention of the APA. I asked whether he saw a high incidence of sexual abuse in his borderline patients. 'Oh yes, I see it all the time,' he said, 'And I have no idea what to make of it.' And then he turned to the next question" (Cauwels 1992, 244). Cauwels interviewed Kernberg about this, and he verified that a review of his data had made him newly aware of the significance of trauma. "'I have changed my views about this matter'" (244).

Judith Herman notes that the pendulum of attention to sexual abuse in borderline patients has now swung the other way, and that it is much more recognized now. "Sexual abuse has been taboo, repressed for so long that it is now entering our consciousness in a very dialectical, polarized way. It has to. If it threatens establishment views, it should, because therapists have really missed the boat in an important way, one that was predictable in a male-dominated profession with a female patient population" (Herman in Cauwels 1992, 250).

For Herman, the borderline's relations to other people can be understood as strategies of adaptation held over from past relations with abusive caretakers:

> Why would a child fail to integrate idealized or terrifying
> images of her caretakers? The reason would have to be either
> constitutional or adaptive. Splitting is adaptive. Children must
> preserve some sense of connection at any cost, in this case by
> walling off the image of the abusive figure from the positive
> one. I think they do so in a state-dependent way, flipping
> between modes of affection and terror that accurately reflect
> their environments. They grow up constantly scanning their
> interpersonal environments to see if they're safe, reading
> subtleties of expression, posture, gesture, and so forth in an
> almost uncanny way. But if you ignore the original reason for
> this behavior, it looks perverse, incomprehensible, and ulti-
> mately pathological. (247)

For Herman, then, trauma provides a narrative comprehensibility to the variety of symptoms expressed by women diagnosed borderline. The patient's instability becomes understood as a response to an external event, rather then being rooted in a character or personality disorder.

And yet the label "borderline personality disorder" lacks such narrative comprehensibility, placing the patient's symptoms within a scientific-medical frame of character pathology. Herman notes the negative effects of this misplaced attention. "Instead of conceptualizing the psychopathology of the victim as a response to an abusive situation, mental health professionals have frequently attributed the abusive situation to the victim's presumed underlying psychopathology" (Herman 1992, 116).

One of Herman's patients, a survivor of sexual abuse, notes the effect of being diagnosed as borderline. "Having that diagnosis [borderline disorder] resulted in my getting treated exactly the way I was treated at home. The minute I got that diagnosis people stopped treating me as though what I was doing had a reason" (128).

To be sure, sexual abuse is a crucial aspect to consider as one of the central aspects of the gender specificity of the disorder. Indeed, this is one of the factors that is neglected in the case narratives as a meaningful aspect of women's suffering. In chapter 5, I examine how the analyst's tendency to minimize the importance of such experience operates to enable the analyst to attribute women's rage and resistance, particularly that aimed at men who are abusive to them, to the deficiencies of their unstable selves. In the language of the narrative approach, we might say that the analyst has missed the patients' story, and so their symptoms appear to lack coherence or meaning.

And yet while sexual abuse is a major factor, it does not fully account for the predominance of women diagnosed as borderline, since not all borderlines have histories of childhood sexual abuse. Becker points out that 20 to 40 percent of women diagnosed as borderline do not have such a background (Becker 1997, 78). Thus, Becker notes, "If BPD cannot be specifically linked only to sexual abuse, then we must develop a broader framework for understanding how women come to be the majority of those diagnosed 'borderline.' There has been much impressive work that has helped us to conceptualize how a sexually abused woman could develop features of borderline personality disorder, but there has been less work aimed specifically at addressing the 'woman question' in the borderline diagnosis" (xv).

Becker sees the feminization of the borderline category as having occurred through a process similar to that of hysteria. While it is not difficult to see the female specificity of hysteria, since it was tied conceptually to the vagaries of the female sexual organs (from the "wandering wombs" of Plato to the "uterine disease" of late-nineteenth-century physicians), Becker focuses on its mutability of symptomatology in comparing it to the borderline category. For both hysteria and borderline, the number and type of symptoms expanded over time, so that it was being applied to more and more women for various ailments. Becker also points to the way in which a central defining feature of the disorders gradually diminished in importance, thus making its meaning more diffuse. For hysteria, this core symptom was the hysterical seizure, a physical episode or "fit" that was similar to an epileptic seizure. Yet this gradually began to decline in the late nineteenth century as a significant feature of hysteria. As Carroll Smith-Rosenberg writes, "By the last third of the nineteenth century the seizure was no longer the central phenomenon defining hysteria; physicians had categorized hysterical symptoms which included virtually every known human ill" (Smith-Rosenberg 1972, 662).

For borderline disorder, the core symptom was brief psychotic symptoms or cognitive distortions (which had placed it on the border with schizophrenia). With the eventual omission of these core symptoms, both hysteria and borderline "came to be signifiers for a heterogeneous group of symptoms that could not easily be said to describe a unitary diagnostic entity" (Becker 1997, 20). Thus, what characterizes the use of borderline disorder and what makes it similar to hysteria is the expansion of symptoms into a catchall or wastebasket category, a flexible diagnosis for a variety of stereotypically female behaviors.

In addition to this expansion of meaning, Becker argues that the diagnosis, in its shifting inclusion of various features and traits, has been feminized in its very meaning. In the last two decades, notes Becker, descriptions of borderline symptoms have moved away from "schizophrenic-like features" and toward traits that stress emotions or affects such as "rage, depression, self-destructiveness (including suicidality), feelings of emptiness and emotional lability" (60). What is significant in this shift away from cognition and toward emotion, argues Becker, is that it is a shift from the more stereotypically "masculine" features and toward more feminine ones, particularly depression, which is more common in women than it is in men.

Becker's observation would seem to be borne out by a comment made by Otto Kernberg in an interview with Janice Cauwels. Kernberg notes that the DSM definition was more narrowly conceived than his more broadly defined category of borderline personality disorder and further, was conceived by a psychiatrist working with women patients. "There are as many males as females with BPO [Borderline Personality Organization], and they are moved into one or another personality constellation by the cultural expression of their symptoms. BPD was described [by Dr. Gunderson] primarily in women hospitalized at McLean, so it picked up one dominant manifestation of severe pathology" (Kernberg, in Cauwels 1992, 143).

In the development of the DSM-III categories, the personality disorders were subdivided into "clusters" that defined their major characteristics; borderline personality disorder is one of the disorders belonging to Cluster B, the "dramatic emotional, erratic group," which also includes narcissistic, histrionic (previously hysterical) and antisocial personality. While some members of the APA task force that developed these category clusters believed they had meaningfully separated qualitatively different types of personality disorder, others felt the categories were arbitrary. Theodore Millon stated that "he never quite understood the importance of those dimensions that led us to cluster personality disorders in the manner described" (Cauwels 1992, 61). However, he writes that "the Borderline personality was formulated to be a disintegrated Dependent, Histrionic, and Passive-aggressive mix, in which the individual's personal cohesion and interpersonal competence were insidiously deteriorated" (Millon 1983, 812).

What is significant in Millon's "disintegrated mix" is that it includes as ingredients two predominantly "female maladies": dependent personality disorder (a style of extreme passivity and reliance on others, more commonly diagnosed in women) and hysteria (histrionic personality disorder). Some psychiatrists have acknowledged this gender-specificity of the definition. Joel Paris, interviewed in Janice Cauwels's book, states, "It's as if whoever wrote the definition had females in mind" (Cauwels 1992, 143).

Under Becker's analysis, then, the codification of borderline diagnosis into a personality disorder in the DSM in 1980 not only marked the medicalization and codification of an unstable personality structure, but also codified a specifically feminized diagnosis. The removal of its association with the border of schizophrenia had the effect of further emphasizing feminine traits.

Further, there is evidence that hysteria in its present guise, histrionic personality disorder, is similar enough to borderline personality disorder that patients could receive either diagnosis. Becker cites a study in which half of subjects in a research group who met the criteria for either one of the disorders also met the criteria for the other (Becker 1997, 59).

While hysteria and borderline categories share a mutability of meaning and a focus on instability, the borderline diagnosis has other, more specific features, that Mary Ann Jimenez believes reflect contemporary gender contradictions. Jimenez notes that during the 1960s and 1970s, hysteria reemerged as a prominent category within a "psychological model" of women's mental illness that replaced the largely biological theories of the late nineteenth and early twentieth centuries. Interest in the "hysterical character" reemerged in the mid 1960s, which Jimenez relates to changes in gender roles. "The reintroduction of hysteria signaled an effort to return to a more traditional conception of women's roles in the face of profound and often unsettling changes in gender relationships" (Jimenez 1997, 157). In the second Diagnostic and Statistical Manual, hysteria was defined as, what Chesler called, "over conformity" to femininity, "essentially a caricature of exaggerated femininity," with "excitability, emotional instability, over-reactivity and self-dramatization" (APA 1968, 251, cited in Jimenez 1997, 158). Jimenez points out moral judgment lay at the heart of the diagnosis, particularly in its attention to "excessive and manipulative sexuality" of the hysterical woman (158).

During the 1970s, interest in hysteria (or histrionic personality disorder, as it was called in the DSM-III) declined. One study showed that after being the third most-discussed category in 1975 (16 percent of psychiatric journal articles) the category fell into relative obscurity in 1985, "not a relatively frequently discussed disorder" (Blashfield and McElroy 1987, 542). Jimenez notes that when hysteria declined as a common label for women's disorders in the early 1980s, borderline diagnosis emerged as a contemporary substitute. "Borderline personality disorder replaced hysteria as the diagnosis that captured contemporary values about appropriate behavior for women" (Jimenez 1997, 161). In part, this may reflect simply a relabeling of the same phenomena under a new category. Judith Herman observes that borderline personality disorder, along with somatization disorder and multiple personality disorder, were once subsumed under the term "hysteria" (Herman 1992, 123). But Jimenez argues that changes in gender roles led to a revision of psychiatric norms regarding appropriate behavior for women. This new successor to hysteria depicted the borderline patient as a "demanding, aggressive, and angry woman" (Jimenez 1997, 162). Jimenez cites a 1990 study (Sprock, Blashfield, and Smith 1990) that found that all of the diagnostic criteria for borderline disorder were judged by clinicians to be "feminine qualities" except for "inappropriate, intense anger," which was viewed as a masculine attribute. Jimenez concludes, "The findings of that study suggest that women who become as angry as men may be considered mentally disordered. A further bias lies in the fact that inappropriate anger is a judgment that is more likely to be made about women than men, because the possibilities for socially legitimate anger are far broader for men" (Jimenez 1997, 163).

Concern with excessive sexuality is another feature of borderline personality disorder, signaling a renewed interest in this "hysterical" trait. Jimenez notes that the concern with sexual promiscuity is evidence of a reaction to women's liberation from traditional sexual norms and reflects a moral judgment of women's transgression of traditional feminine roles: "The concept of borderline personality disorder is rooted in a moral vision of what constitutes mentally healthy behavior; the timeliness of its emergence in a period of growing flexibility in gender roles and greater choices and diversity in potential lifestyles demonstrates its salience as a modern successor to hysteria" (165–166). When coupled with another personality disorder, dependent personality disorder, also newly introduced into the DSM-III in 1980, the borderline diagnosis defines one end of a "psychological-moral ideology to bracket acceptable behavior for women, just as hysteria offered women of earlier eras normative guideposts . . . These personality disorders define the mentally healthy woman as one who is renewed and energized by social change and no longer dependent on men, but neither angry nor aggressive" (167).

Taken together, the analyses of Becker, Herman, and Jimenez provide a helpful framework for considering the relation of gender norms and meanings to the borderline diagnosis, and situates its emergence within post-1960s changes in women's social positioning. These changes are important to understand as the context within which women's identities or selves are perceived as unstable.

The evidence does suggest that it is in the more recent manifestations that the borderline category becomes fully feminized, and the predominance of women becomes more visible here. However, a close look at case narratives reveals the feminine connotations of the borderline category prior to its entrance in the DSM-III. In the analysis of case narratives, I will show that some of the roots of the current predominance of women among those diagnosed borderline may be traced to these earlier cases, in which the borderline diagnosis is linked to unstable self-identity, unstable emotions, and anger that is defined as inappropriate or excessive. It might be said that certain discursive associations of the borderline concept with femininity which appear in the case narratives were codified when the diagnosis was made official in the DSM.

Men and Borderline Instability

Another avenue for exploring the feminization of the borderline category is to explore the instances when men receive the diagnosis. Men are in the minority of patients receiving this diagnosis; roughly 25 percent to 30 percent of those diagnosed as borderline are males (Becker 1997, xxii). One of the main explanations offered for the low numbers of men diagnosed as borderline is that males showing similar traits as borderline women tend to be diagnosed as sociopathic, or as having antisocial personality disorder (Cauwels 1192, 143). According to this view, some male patients may express the same confusion and uncertainty or instability and rage as women, but tend to direct their rage toward others, rather than toward themselves. Thus, they become involved with the legal system, rather than the mental health system. Noting that a large proportion (25 percent) of patients with antisocial personality disorder also fulfill the criteria for borderline personality disorder, Gunderson and Zanarini write, "Sex bias probably prejudices clinicians to overlook the antisocial features of female patients and the dependent, needy (borderline) features of male patients" (Gunderson and Zanarini 1987, 7).

Other psychiatrists disagree, arguing that antisocial personality disorder is not the same as borderline personality disorder, in that it does not include the fluctuating emotions described in borderline disorders. Larry J. Siever comments, "I think that antisocial personality disorder is not the same as BPD because it's missing the affective component. Most borderline patients seek clinical treatment because they are depressed. I think that much of the male equivalent of borderlines may be as close—or closer—to narcissistic as to antisocial personality disorders" (Siever, in Cauwels 1992, 143).

Significantly, a high proportion of the men who do receive the diagnosis of borderline are said to be homosexual. Joel Paris states, "It has been shown that a larger percentage of male borderlines than we would expect are homosexual, and that's interesting" (Paris, in Cauwels 1992, 143). One question bearing on this pattern is whether women and gay men express similar kinds of identity disturbances that are said to be characteristic of the borderline patient; or whether this pattern is an outcome of clinicians perceiving, and hence labeling them in similar ways.

A clinical supervisor at a Boston-area counseling center has observed that borderline patients she has treated frequently experience ambivalence and confusion over their sexual identity. She states that the majority of male borderline patients she has treated have been homosexual or bisexual, and that much of their treatment centers on sexual identity and gender identity conflicts. Because sexual/gender identity is so pivotal to a person's sense of self, the identity and self-fragmentation that characterizes borderline disorder frequently becomes a struggle over gender or sexual identity. Often this is complicated by a history of sexual abuse. This counselor provided the example of one male patient who entered treatment to overcome feelings of shame associated with denigration he had experienced from others, including an incident of sexual abuse from an older boy in his school.

Clinicians' perception of the outward expressions of borderline patients may be another level at which commonalties exist between women and men diagnosed as borderline. The authors of one study found that an approximately equal number of Hispanic men as Hispanic women were diagnosed as borderline, and they suggest that this may be due to Hispanic men's greater degree of emotional expressivity, more accepted in Hispanic cultures, as compared to African American or Caucasian men (Castaneda and Franco 1985, 10). There may be a similar process of gendered emotional experience and expressivity occurring for homosexual men. Yet this raises the question of the cultural perception of such emotional expressivity in men. Castaneda and Franco suggest that Hispanic men's exuberance may be perceived and labeled as deviant by the predominantly white psychiatric establishment. Again, this raises the question of whether homosexual men's emotional expression of psychic or identity conflicts is perceived as mental pathology by a predominantly heterosexual white male psychiatric/psychoanalytic institution. This echoes the history of psychoanalytic perception of homosexuality as neurosis, with those labeled borderline manifesting more severe personality disturbances than their oedipally disturbed counterparts.

Other evidence suggests overall, men may escape the label of borderline because most of their expressions of borderlinelike behaviors are viewed as appropriate to the masculine gender role, and hence not signs of pathology. A study of respondents in the general population who answered a questionnaire that measured borderline symptoms found that men in the general population reported more borderline characteristics than normal women. The authors conclude that this is evidence for the influence of gender bias in labeling women in clinical settings. "Given that normal men report more borderline characteristics than normal women, it is interesting to speculate that clinicians may consider these characteristics as more congruent with male sex roles and may find them more tolerable in men. Conversely, in women these traits may be seen as less appropriate to sex role, and therefore women may be more likely to be labeled as having borderline personality disorder" (Henry and Cohen 1983, 1529).

In *Women and Madness*, Phyllis Chesler writes, "What we consider 'madness,' whether it appears in women or in men, is either the acting out of the devalued female role or the total or partial rejection of one's sex-role stereotype" (Chesler 1989, 56). Men who "act out the devalued feminine role" Chesler notes, and who " are 'dependent,' 'passive,' sexually and physically 'fearful' or 'inactive,' or who, like women, choose men as sexual partners, are seen as 'neurotic' or 'psychotic.' (57). On the other hand, men who "act out the male role," "but who are too young, too poor, or too black—are usually incarcerated as 'criminals' or as 'sociopaths,' rather than as 'schizophrenics' or 'neurotics.'" (57). The evidence briefly discussed here on the borderline diagnosis bears out this pattern of gender specificity in the labeling of women and men mentally ill. Men who are diagnosed as borderline are those who deviate from the masculine gender stereotype. Chapter 3 explores this pattern in more detail in an examination of male cases that focus on lapses in proper masculinity. Yet it also discusses cases of males who appear to "act out the male role" in their behavior and yet who receive the borderline diagnosis. However, an examination of the cases shows that, unlike women, these males are not defined as unstable.

Conclusion

Psychiatrists and psychoanalysts have struggled to represent the nebulous region between sanity and madness, a terrain that has captured the psychiatric imagination since the nineteenth century. Between the early conception of the borderland, to the listing of symptoms for the unstable personality in the DSM, the concept of borderline has been defined in multiple ways. During the nineteenth century, the concept of the borderland referred to a region inhabited by those socially wayward individuals thought to be afflicted with hereditary taint; the emergence of psychoanalysis in U.S. psychiatry saw the psychoanalytic construction of the borderline between psychosis (schizophrenia) and neurosis; and finally, the contemporary psychiatric definition of the borderline personality disorder, within the DSM-III, characterized by instability. Within the parameters of these broad trends, the meaning of the concept, and the definition of the kind of patient designated as borderline, have remained elusive. The purported instability of the borderline patient is reflected in the unstable and shifting meanings of the term through its conceptual history.

Yet in spite of this ambiguity, psychiatric and psychoanalytic discourse has succeeded in constructing a hegemonic meaning for the term, asserting that clearly defined borders exist and can be identified for the borderline personality. This culminates in the borderline category's entrance into the DSM. The earlier uncertainty and controversy has been smoothed over with this standardized definition.

Yet as the discussion by Reiser and Levenson of the derogatory uses of the borderline diagnosis shows, in spite of this imposed consensus, the term continues to be used in multiple ways, often with pejorative overtones. The borderline diagnosis is often used as a wastebasket category, where those persons whom psychoanalysts cannot classify in the existing categories are placed.

The feminization of the borderline category is exemplified in the evidence for Becker's and Jimenez's claim that the borderline category is a contemporary successor to hysteria. Becker's analysis illuminates the similarities between borderline and hysteria, showing that, like hysteria, the borderline diagnosis has expanded into an overinclusive and diffuse category. Moreover, its use as a derogatory label for the troublesome female patient is also analogous to the nineteenth-century usage of hysteria. Jimenez argues that the borderline label represents new cultural norms for feminine behavior in reaction to women's assertiveness and anger, norms that then translate into psychiatric definitions of mental pathology.

Another aspect of the feminization of the borderline is the large number of borderline patients with histories of sexual abuse. For Herman, the symptoms that come to be grouped under the label of borderline represent patterns of adaptation to abuse, rather than an underlying personality disorder. Herman's reframing of borderline symptoms is crucial in providing a contextual meaning for women's behavior that is deemed unstable. These women's ways of acting are made comprehensible as responses to an external event, and moreover, an event located in gender relations of power. The coming chapters examine the importance of abuse and violence as a crucial context for the emergence of women's symptoms labeled borderline. And yet, as Becker argues, the gender connotations of borderline disorder go beyond the specific issue of sexual abuse, requiring a broader study of the "woman question" in the borderline. These chapters also examine other dimensions of gender that contribute to the feminization of the borderline label, including the discursive connotations of instability as culturally allied to the feminine and the symbolic and cultural position of woman as Other to dominant conceptions of selfhood.

Chapter 3

Women on the Borders

Feminine Instability

Societies do not succeed in offering everyone the same way of fitting into the symbolic order; those who are, if one may say so, between symbolic systems, in the interstices, offsides, are the ones who are afflicted with a dangerous symbolic mobility. Dangerous for them, because those are the people afflicted with what we call madness, anomaly, perversion . . . And more than any others, women bizarrely embody this group of anomalies showing the cracks in an overall system.

(Clément 1986, 7)

Women's social or cultural marginality seems to place them on the borderline of the symbolic order, both the "frontier between men and chaos" and dangerously part of chaos itself, inhabitants of a mysterious and frightening wild zone outside of patriarchal culture.

(Showalter 1990, 4)

CATHERINE CLÉMENT'S COMMENT comes in the context of a discussion of the role of the hysteric in culture in the book *The Newly Born Women* (Cixous and Clément 1986). Clément draws on Lévi-Strauss's structural analysis of women's position in the sex-gender system, as an object of exchange in patriarchal culture, and yet as an "anomaly" in the cultural order. Like the mad, and like the "neurotics, ecstatics, outsiders, carnies, drifters, jugglers and acrobats," in the words of Marcel Mauss, women are positioned "in the interstices" of the cultural order, since by virtue of their bodies, they are located at the boundaries between nature and culture. Lévi-Strauss's analysis, Clément writes, suggests that "Women . . . are double. They are allied with what is regular, according to the rules, since they are wives and mothers, and allied as well with those natural disturbances, their regular periods, which are the epitome of paradox, order and disorder. It is precisely in this natural periodicity that fear, terror, that which is offside in the symbolic system will lodge itself. Michelet was right: the sorceress conceives Nature, and woman, the periodic being, takes part in something that is not contained within culture" (Clément 1986, 8).

It is this contradictory position of women in the cultural order that forms the context for this examination of the representation of women deemed borderline. The borderline is said to lack a stable, coherent self. And yet women's relationship to dominant conceptions of self and identity is complex. Self and identity are not only historically constructed concepts that may function as regulatory ideals in a culture, but are also constructed within the hierarchical sex-gender system. The binary logic of gender discourse creates a powerful matrix of meaning within which individuals take up positions of identity and construct narratives of selfhood. Women's complex relation to this logic of identity is discussed here, in order to provide a context for analyzing how, in the case narratives of borderline patients, certain women patients are depicted as lacking stable selfhood. How does the cultural position of women "in the interstices, offsides"—in short, on the borders of the cultural order— condition the representation of certain women patients as borderline?

In this chapter, I outline a feminist critique of the representation of femininity in Western culture, focusing on the construction of woman as Other in relation to the autonomous, self-defined subject. More than simply a linguistic convention or bias, this representation of women has a material basis in women's position in relation to the cultural order as the object of exchange in sex-gender marriage systems (Irigaray 1985; Rubin 1975).

I then examine how this construction of woman as Other appears in psychoanalytic discourse in depictions of women as unstable and mutable. Because borderline disorder is a contemporary successor to hysteria, I briefly discuss the association of hysteria with feminine instability. Next, I explore the feminine connotations of instability in the case narratives of borderline patients. While hysteria was defined as an emotional lability and capriciousness, the borderline's instability is depicted as a more threatening formlessness of the self. The borderline patient is depicted as uncanny, unwilling to interact in comprehensible ways during therapy sessions, thus putting the patient's very coherence as a subject in question.

Woman as Other

The category of "woman" in Western representational systems stands in a precarious and unstable place in relation to the humanist ideal of a generic, neutral, universal "subject"—the Western "self-defining subject" (Sass 1988). The feminist critique of this subject asserts that it is gendered, conceptualized as inherently masculine. "Woman" is represented as Other to this ideal of the universal subject, and women's specific experiences are excluded from, or defined in negative opposition to, that purportedly neutral subject.

Many feminist analyses draw on Lévi-Strauss's analysis of the exchange of women to articulate women's position in the cultural order (Butler 1990; de Lauretis 1984; Irigaray 1985; Rubin 1975). Lévi-Strauss showed that in cultures built on gift exchange, women, along with other valuable gifts ("food, spells, rituals, words, names, ornaments, tools, and powers" [Rubin 1975, 171]) are the most precious of gifts within the basic exchange of marriage. According to Lévi-Strauss, marriage is an exchange that adheres to the prohibition of the incest taboo, and insures that exchanges take place between kin groups. The exchange of a sister or daughter in marriage establishes, not just an exchange relation of reciprocity, but a kinship relation, a relation of blood. Further, this exchange is guaranteed by the patronym, the authority of the father in patrilineal descent. Hence women, in Lévi-Strauss's theory, become central as exchange to the foundation of culture.

A woman in this exchange assumes the status of gift, object exchanged, and not that of subject who exchanges. Women, with no gift to give, no "rights of bestowal" of other women, "are in no position to give themselves away" (Rubin 175). Thus women are located in the interstices of social exchange, off-center from subjecthood, serving as the medium of exchange between subjects. The position of woman functions as "a relational term between groups of men; she does not have an identity . . . she reflects masculine identity precisely through being the site of its absence" (Butler 1990, 39).

Yet Lévi-Strauss recognized that women are not simply exchange objects, but "even in a man's world she is still a person, and since in so far as she is defined as a sign she must be recognized as a generator of signs" (Lévi-Strauss 1969, 496). Jacques Lacan comments on women's "impossible" position, stating, "That the woman should be inscribed in an order of exchange of which she is the object, is what makes for the fundamentally conflictual, and I would say, insoluble, character of her position: the symbolic order literally submits her, it transcends her. . . . There is for her something insurmountable, something unacceptable, in the fact of being placed as an object in a symbolic order to which, at the same time, she is subjected just as much as the man" (Lacan, in Mitchell and Rose 1982, 45).

For Catherine Clément, this ambiguous and unstable position is a "stress point" in the cultural logic, a place where meaning is mobile and shifting, thus revealing the instability of the cultural order. Women are "afflicted with a dangerous symbolic mobility . . . showing the cracks in an overall system." Jane Gallop comments on this dual status of women as both subject and object. "Woman's ambiguous cultural place may be precisely the standpoint from which it is possible to muddle the sub-ject/object distinction, that distinction necessary for a certain episte-mological relation to the world" (Gallop 1985, 15).

Just as they are materially positioned as Other in the logic of ex-change, women are ideologically rendered as Other in language. Many feminist analyses draw upon Derrida's critique of the logic of identity to articulate women's position in language. For Derrida, Western sys-tems of meaning are built on a binary logic that is both dualistic and hierarchical. Language is constructed based on pairs of opposite terms, which are defined in a hierarchical relation in which one term is as-sumed to be primary and superior (mind, spirit, light) while the other is figured as secondary, inferior, and derivative (body, matter, dark). Bi-nary logic serves to "subordinate these values to each other (normal/abnormal, standard/parasite, fulfilled/void, serious/non-serious, literal/non-literal, briefly: positive/negative and ideal/non-ideal" (Derrida, quoted in Ryan 1982, 10).

Hence identity is defined through difference, and something ac-quires its meaning through its difference from what is excluded as de-rivative and of lesser value. And the feminist analysis argues that the dominant Western conceptions of the subject—the self-defined, unified, and autonomous subject—was constructed through its repression of the feminine. Hélène Cixous writes, "Organization by hierarchy makes all conceptual organization subject to man. Male privilege, shown in the opposition between activity and passivity, which he uses to sustain himself. Traditionally, the question of sexual difference is treated by coupling it with the opposition: activity/passivity. . . . Moreover, woman is always associated with passivity in philosophy" (Cixous and Clément 1986, 64).

The hierarchical value of mind and reason over the body is most explicitly articulated in Descartes's philosophy, which makes a rigid distinction between subject and object, creating the illusion of an autonomous, free-willed subject, in control of the observable world, and able to transcend the limits of nature and of the body. Susan Bordo analyzes Descartes's *Méditations* as a reflection of the seventeenth century's central anxieties. Bordo notes that Descartes's scheme inaugurates a world in which a "clear and distinct sense of the boundaries of the self has become the ideal." Descartes's stance, in which the senses of the body are ignored in favor of pure objective reason ("I shall close my eyes, I shall stop my ears, I shall call away all my senses") results in "a securing of all the boundaries that, in childhood, are so fragile: between the 'inner' and the 'outer,' between the subjective and the objective, between self and world" (Bordo 1986, 450). "For Descartes, an epistemological chasm separates a highly self-conscious self from a universe that now lies decisively outside the self" resulting in a "profound Cartesian experience of self as inwardness ('I think, therefore I am') and its corollary—the heightened sense of distance from the 'not-I'" (444).

Within Western philosophy and epistemology, "woman" becomes apprehended as part of the denied separate world. Woman and the feminine are situated on the side of the secondary, inferior, derivative term, constructed as Other to the West's highest values. Here Elaine Showalter's comment regarding the deep symbolic link between cultural ideas of "femininity" and madness is again appropriate: "Women, within our dualistic systems of language and representation, are typically situated on the side of irrationality, silence, nature, and body, while men are situated on the side of reason, discourse, culture and mind" (Showalter 1985, 4).

Thus, in the logic of the gender binary, the category "woman" is positioned as Other, a lack against which the masculine subject defines itself. The universal subject attains substance and meaning only through the exclusion and repression of the feminine. Simone de Beauvoir writes of the effects of this binary logic of gender: "Thus humanity is male and man defines woman not in herself but as relative to him; she is not regarded as an autonomous being. . . . And she is simply what man decrees; thus she is called 'the sex,' by which is meant that she appears essentially to the male as a sexual being. For him she is sex—absolute sex, no less. She is defined and differentiated with reference to man and not he with reference to her; she is the incidental, the inessential as opposed to the essential. He is the Subject, he is the Absolute—she is the Other" (Beauvoir 1989, xxii).

Judith Butler summarizes this position as represented by Simone de Beauvoir: "For Beauvoir, the 'subject' within the existential analytic of misogyny is always already masculine, conflated with the universal, differentiating itself from a feminine 'Other' outside the universalizing norms of personhood, hopelessly 'particular,' embodied, condemned to immanence" (Butler 1990, 11).

Luce Irigaray's conception of the position of "woman" takes Beauvoir's position to its extreme. Irigaray argues that there is only one sex, the masculine, that "elaborates itself in and through the production of the 'Other'" (Butler 1990, 18). As Butler points out: "For Irigaray, the female sex is not a 'lack' or an 'Other' that immanently and negatively defines the subject in its masculinity. On the contrary, the female sex eludes the very requirements of representation, for she is neither 'Other' nor the 'lack,' those categories remaining relative to the Sartrian subject, immanent to that phallogocentric scheme" (10). In other words, the feminine is not a negatively defined derivative or opposite of masculinity, but another version of the same masculine image. Both terms of the binary, the masculine subject and its "other" are different images of masculine identity. The singular masculine model of subjectivity defines itself in woman, using her as mirror image. Irigaray's critique extends to the very conception of a subject, which she argues is itself a "masculinist construction and prerogative which effectively excludes the structural and semantic possibility of a feminine gender" (11).

This leads to Irigaray's conclusions regarding woman in this logic: "Unconsciousness she is, but not for herself, not with a subjectivity that might take cognizance of it, recognize it as her own. Close to herself, admittedly, but in a total ignorance (of self). She is the reserve of 'sensuality' for the elevation of intelligence, she is the matter used for the imprint of forms, gage of possible regression into naive perception, the representative representing negativity (death), dark continent of dreams and fantasies, and also eardrum faithfully duplicating the music, though not all of it, so that the series of displacements may continue, for the 'subject'" (Irigaray 1985, 141).

The implications of these analyses of women's impossible borderline position are critical to the consideration of representation of women as subject, particularly when that subjecthood is said to be unstable or lacking. The cultural logic that situates women in this unstable, intermediary position operates as a powerful constraint on what women are allowed to be, how they are represented in discourse, and how they represent themselves. The autonomous universal subject gains its identity through the suppression and exclusion of feminine difference. For theorists such as Beauvoir, the place of woman is inhabited by the devalued projections of Western masculinist culture, a negative status, a lack. Women are defined as the derivative of the subject. For Irigaray, woman is condemned to masquerade as a cultural projection.

Here the concept of the "abject" is helpful in understanding exclusion of difference and the threat posed by that difference. The abject is a concept developed by Julia Kristeva, who draws from Mary Douglas's work on how social and cultural boundaries become inscribed in ideas about bodily boundaries. The abject is that which is excluded from the body in order to demarcate it as a bounded, homogeneous, and coherent entity. As Judith Butler describes it, "the 'abject' designates that which has been expelled from the body, discharged as excrement, literally rendered 'Other.' . . . The construction of the 'not-me' as the abject establishes the boundaries of the body which are also the first contours of the subject" (Butler 1990, 133).

Butler appropriates the concept of "abjection" to foreground society's exclusion of certain social identities in order to maintain the illusion of the dominant coherent, self-identical subject (Herman 1999, 85). Naming "is at once the setting of a boundary, and also the repeated inculcation of a norm"; and such instances of social boundary marking "contribute to that field of discourse and power that orchestrates, de-limits, and sustains that which qualifies as 'the human'" (Butler 1993, 8). Abject beings, then, are not afforded the status of the human, or coherence of selfhood.

Yet the boundaries demarcating the coherent subject are permeable, and thus the realm of the Other threatens to leak back across the bor-ders of the subject and contaminate it. Hence the abject is dangerous, threatening, even horrifying. As Elizabeth Grosz notes, it is the abject's very location on the borderline between inner and outer, self and not-self, that makes it threatening, because it remains irreducible to either subject/object, or inside/outside. "The Abject necessarily partakes of both polarized terms but cannot be clearly identified with either" (Grosz 1994, 192). Further, the abject is frequently represented as a dangerous and contaminating fluidity. "Douglas refers to all borderline states, func-tions, and positions as danger, sites of possible pollution or contamina-tion. That which is marginal is always located as a site of danger and vulnerability. She, like Kristeva, conceives of the fluid as a borderline state, disruptive of the solidity of things, entities, and objects" (195).

Grosz notes that fluidity is symbolically associated with feminin-ity, and that both are viewed with a kind of horror:

> It is the production of an order that renders female sexuality
> and corporeality marginal, indeterminate, and viscous that
> constitutes the sticky and the viscous with their disgusting,
> horrifying connotations. Irigaray claims that this disquiet about
> the fluid, the viscous, the half-formed, or the indeterminate has
> to do with the cultural unrepresentability of fluids within
> prevailing philosophical models of ontology, their implicit
> association with femininity, with maternity, with the corporeal,
> all elements subordinated to the privilege of the self-identical,
> the one, the unified, the solid. (195)

Here I explore the ways certain female patients deemed borderline are said to occupy this space of the abject. If the unified, coherent self is the "regulatory ideal," the "unity, the essence, the existential core, and the mastermind of one's life," in Schafer's words, patients who come to be labeled as borderline are defined against this ideal as incoherent, lacking a unified self. Thus, the borderline as a signifier comes to refer not simply to the location between neurosis and psychosis, but to this indeterminate, and therefore threatening, position of abjection. This incoherence is narrativized, in the depictions of the patients' outward appearance, incomprehensible actions, and responses to the analytic situation. Most important, the unstable self is described and interpreted in relation to dominant meanings of femininity itself as unstable.

In the case narratives, this unstable and incoherent abjection is depicted as a space of chaos, inhumanness, or danger. The borderline diagnosis is applied to certain women patients who are difficult, who resist the work of therapy, or who are socially marginal. Frequently the case narrative of the borderline patient centers on the patient's transgression of boundaries—of the therapeutic relationship, of the rituals of behavior during therapy, or social boundaries such as sexuality, dress, or the appropriate expression of emotion. The narratives depict the patient as excessive, raging, uncontrolled, or manipulative. These abject borderlines are threatening to the analyst, not only because they pose the danger of the feminine, abject not-self, but also because they destabilize the therapeutic situation. The instability and chaos of analysts' turbulent interactions with borderlines, however, is projected onto the borderline as an inner mental pathology, a structural instability of self.

Before discussing the borderline case narratives, I will briefly examine the theme of instability in the historical meanings of hysteria. If the borderline category is the contemporary successor to hysteria as a label for female disorder, it is important to examine how the meanings of instability and femininity were historically linked in the definition of hysteria.

Hysteria and Instability: A Capricious Femininity

The contemporary association of femininity with instability in depictions of borderline conditions can be traced by examining the theme of instability in hysteria. As Showalter notes, during the "Golden Era" of hysteria, from 1870 to World War I, it assumed a "peculiarly central role in psychiatric discourse, and in definitions of femininity and female sexuality," so much so that by the end of the century, "'hysterical' had become almost interchangeable with 'feminine' in literature, where it stood for all extremes of emotionality" (Showalter 1985, 129).

One of the defining features of hysteria, and one that seems to capture an essential quality of femininity at the heart of its meaning, is mutability, instability, or capriciousness, all qualities that were also defining features of femininity. Carroll Smith-Rosenberg writes that "for centuries hysteria has been seen as the embodiment of a perverse or hyper femininity" (Smith-Rosenberg 1972, 653). Hysteria, writes Susan Bordo, represented an exaggeration of a nineteenth century ideal of "a charmingly labile and capricious emotionality" (16). One physician, Dr. Edward J. Tilt, stated in 1881 that "mutability is characteristic of hysteria, because it is characteristic of women—'La donna è mobile'" (Tilt 1881, cited in Showalter 1985, 129).

This preoccupation with feminine mutability can be traced to the beliefs about feminine physiology that predominated during the nineteenth century. The vagaries of women's reproductive cycle, from menarche and puberty to childbirth and menopause, made them especially vulnerable to nervous disease. Further, deviant feminine sexuality was suspected as the cause of hysteria, whether it be through masturbation, sex outside of marriage, or even an excessive sexuality inside it (Smith-Rosenberg 1972, 670). Smith-Rosenberg notes that the hysteric was described as having lost control over her mind and body, and hence was more likely to succumb to "morbid" thoughts. "Such women were described as weak, capricious and, perhaps most important, morbidly suggestible" (Smith-Rosenberg 1972, 668).

When the seizure declined in significance as a defining feature of the hysteria in the late nineteenth century, attention to the "hysterical character" or "hysterical personality" began to rise to prominence. "An hysterical female character gradually began to emerge in the nineteenth-century medical literature, one based on interpretations of mood and personality rather than on discrete physical symptoms—one which grew closely to resemble twentieth-century definitions of the 'hysterical personality.' Doctors commonly described hysterical women as highly impressionistic, suggestible, and narcissistic. Highly labile, their moods changed suddenly, dramatically, and for seemingly inconsequential reasons" (Smith-Rosenberg 1972, 662).

While hysteria declined as a focus of attention during the twentieth century, there was a surge of renewed attention to the "hysterical personality" between 1964 and 1975 (Jimenez 1997, 156). Again the definition focuses on instability. As defined in 1968, in the second edition of the Diagnostic and Statistical Manual of Mental Disorders, the hysterical personality is characterized by "excitability, emotional instability, overreactivity, self-dramatization, attention seeking, immaturity, vanity, and unusual dependence" (Lazare 1971, 131). Beyond this official definition, the term, like the borderline label, was also used as a term of denigration, as Aaron Lazare wrote of its "non-psychoanalytic uses": "'Hysterical' is commonly used in a pejorative sense to describe a patient who is self-engrossed, incapable of loving deeply, lacking depth, emotionally shallow, fraudulent in affect, immature, emotionally incontinent, and a great liar" (Lazare 1971, 131).

Even in its more recent version, histrionic personality disorder, hysteria is defined in stereotypically feminine ways. As Marcie Kaplan notes, the symptoms of histrionic personality disorder (including self-dramatization, exaggerated expression of emotions; irrational, angry outbursts or tantrums, being vain and demanding; and dependent, helpless, constantly seeking reassurance) overlap with the biases found in the Broverman study regarding so-called normal adult females. "It appears then that via assumptions about sex roles made by clinicians, a healthy woman automatically earns the diagnosis of Histrionic Personality Disorder" (Kaplan 1983, 789).

During the period when hysteria was declining in significance as a common diagnostic category, borderline personality disorder was emerging as a prominent female diagnosis. Jimenez argues that this new successor to hysteria, in depicting the borderline patient as a "demanding, aggressive, and angry woman" (Jimenez 1997, 162), and in highlighting as one of its features "promiscuity" in sexuality, is reflective of contemporary moral judgments of normal female behavior, in a climate of changing gender expectations. (163). In the following discussion, I examine the case narratives to trace the contours of this new unstable, aggressive image and to explore the types of women patients who receive this diagnosis.

Describing the "Off-Center" Woman

Borderline disorder is said to be defined by instability: it "not only *causes* instability, but also *symbolizes* it" (Cauwels 1992, 82). As defined in psychiatric discourse, borderline symptoms embody uncertainty and instability: instability in self-image, mood, relationships; feelings of emptiness, indifference, or rage.

Countertransference—the unconscious and conscious emotional responses of the analyst to the patient—is significant as a sign of the analyst's desire, which drives the interpretation and narrative representation of the patient. Freud's countertransference with Dora—his anxiety about its incompleteness and fragmentary status, his feeling of having been "deserted" by Dora, his uncertainty about the scientific status of his work, his unconscious identification with the men in Dora's story, particularly Herr K., all contribute to a field of interpretation that is not neutral as to gender and power.

Countertransference figures prominently in the analysis of borderline patients. One of the major themes in the borderline case narratives is the turbulent relationship between the patient and therapist. The borderline patient has an intense effect on the analyst, and this is frequently attributed to the patient's inconsistent or contradictory behavior in therapy and in outside relationships. Borderline patients resist the role of patient, or reject various aspects of the therapeutic situation. They appear elusive to their analysts, seeming to resist efforts to be defined. Such inconsistency makes the therapeutic relationship itself, and the positions or roles of patient and therapist, highly unstable, thus disrupting the routine of psychiatric interpretation. The emotions and reactions of transference and countertransference become predominant themes in the text, as the psychiatrist relates her or his struggle to define and treat the patient. The transferential relations between therapist and patient are characterized as a struggle over boundaries, with the patient either refusing to play the role of patient, or trying to enter the therapist's personal life.

The borderline patient sometimes has the effect of destabilizing the psychiatrist's certainty and identity, as this example illustrates:

> The borderline personality goes through a far more rapid
> sequence. One day he represents everything as marvelous and
> one is treated as a fine, helpful and most supportive person. The
> next day, one may encounter the borderline individual in his
> "bad" state; the air feels tense; it is hard to breathe; one tends
> to feel insecure. One may talk a lot, or else feel that it's hard to

say anything. It isn't that one feels controlled, as with the narcissistic character. . . . Instead one feels driven to do something, and if we look carefully, that act is generally to survive with a sense of identity. (Schwartz-Salant 1987, 117)

This discomfort evoked by the borderline patient is further described as a sense of being scrutinized by the patient:

Amidst the emotional assaults he may feel—intense experiences that may result in a temporary loss of his sense of identity, wholeness and Eros—he also may tend to feel that the borderline person ("Who is borderline now?" is a question!) knows something. At first experienced as a vague uneasiness, this feeling makes him think he did err or somehow do harm. The patient may be totally unable to verbalize this, instead assaulting the therapist with an unpleasant energy field. The therapist becomes subject to the patient's scanning, a kind of imaginal sight that is peculiarly discomforting. His sight is like the Negative Eye Goddess . . . in ancient Egypt, who roamed the waters before creation, destroying everything she saw. (117)

Yet this destabilization of the situation is managed by attributing it to the patient's mental instability. Psychiatrists look to patients' underlying pathology as an explanatory model for the instability and flux of the situation, thereby making sense of borderline patients' unpredictable behavior. Instability becomes the unity in the otherwise diverse and confusing array of symptoms that a patient who is to be diagnosed as borderline is said to exhibit. This statement illustrates this construction of a unity from fragments: "At some point, however, most clients usually notice that instability itself describes much of their behavior—frequent changes in mood, in sense of identity, and in feelings toward others. Ironically, the perception of a pattern of instability can be itself a stabilizing feature of the borderline. It helps to stimulate, to at least some degree, the sense of continuity through space and time" (De Chenne 1991, 288).

This therapist encourages borderline patients to become aware of their instability and even to learn about their diagnosis, arguing that it fosters an "observing ego" to develop and manage the oscillations of their behavior. It is this elevation of inconsistency to the level of a syndrome that enables therapists to make a diagnosis of borderline personality disorder out of this diverse group.

Frequently one of the first cues in the narrative that therapists present as evidence of an underlying instability is that of outward appearance. Peter Brooks points out that often the opening of a narrative sets it in motion and provides the energy of desire and curiosity for what is to come: "One could no doubt analyze the opening paragraph of most novels and emerge in each case with the image of a desire taking on shape, beginning to seek its objects, beginning to develop a textual energetics" (Brooks 1984, 38).

This is apparent in the opening paragraphs of many case narratives, which begin with a physical description of the patient, to give "first impressions" that provide the mystery of disturbance, and set the narrative in motion toward discovering its causes. The patient may be described as "off-center" in dress, makeup, expression, or mannerisms. This outward incoherence is then understood by the therapist as a sign of an inner incoherence of selfhood, as illustrated by this description of a patient by Irvin Yalom: "She did not belong to herself, nothing went with anything else—her hair, her grin, her voice, her walk, her sweater, her shoes, everything had been flung together by chance, and there was the immediate possibility of all—hair, walk, limbs, tattered jeans, G.I. socks, everything—flying asunder. Leaving what? I wondered. Perhaps just the grin. Not pretty, no matter how one arranged the parts!" (Yalom 1974, xi).

Yalom's image of physical disarray is equated with the image of coherence of selfhood. The focus on appearance, particularly of clothing, hair, and facial expression, as indicative of mental coherence and intelligibility, reproduces a historic theme of the equation of women mental patients' health and progress with attractive appearance (Showalter 1985, 212). And the image of the scattered fragments of Ginny's physical presence being "flung together" or flying apart suggests a definition of mental conflict that concerns not the conflict between two opposing forces, or the contradiction between an outer surface and an internal, secret self; rather, the image is one of a surface clash of disparate elements that don't cohere. The problem is not a self divided against itself, but rather a shattered self, artificially assembled.

In another example, Martin Stein, writing of his first meeting of his patient Ms. V., also equates an outward incoherence with an inner disturbance:

> My initial impression upon meeting this woman was striking. She was of above average height, slightly overweight, and while she had attractive facial features something about her was not quite right, something didn't "fit." Even though her clothing was expensive and fashionable, it never quite fit. The normal nips, tugs and pulls, that one usually does in the morning in front of the mirror was apparently not engaged in by this woman, resulting in her having a rather disoriented, unsymmetrical, and perhaps fragmented appearance. This does not mean that she wasn't neat, rather, I got the impression of a person who was "off center," not in the manner of eccentricity, but rather a reflection of an inner structural disturbance. Even her lipstick appeared to extend slightly above the natural contours of her lips. (Stein 1989, 124)

The analyst goes on to describe Ms. V.'s exaggerated, almost garish feminine appearance, describing her "flaming red lipstick, black eye liner, false eye lashes and hair dyed jet black. . . . At times, she reminded me of the vampire wife of Herman Munster of the television series 'The Munsters,' and at other times of a caricature of Joan Collins of 'Dynasty' fame" (124). Stein's description of this caricatured femininity is central to his interpretation, which comes later; what is important to point out here is the conception of an incoherent "off center," and excessive femininity, coded through visual appearance.

From these initial impressions of an outward incoherence, the narratives move on to describe the patient's unstable and often bewildering behavior. The case narratives often center on the patients' transgression of boundaries both in the rituals of therapy and in the patients' outside life.

The case of Ann, a twenty-two-year old borderline patient, illustrates the theme of the turbulent, unstable therapeutic relationship, as well as how this turbulence is projected onto the patient as borderline pathology (Waldinger and Gunderson 1987). Ann behaves in a manner that breaks the rules of psychotherapy, and she appears to offer resistance to playing the role of patient. This resistance effectively reverses the roles of patient and therapist, with the patient scrutinizing the analyst. This visual scrutiny appears in the opening to the account, with the future patient watching the therapist without his awareness at a funeral for her former psychiatrist. In the first session, Ann behaves in a manner that breaks several rules of the ritual of therapy, as well as rules of everyday interaction. As her therapist writes:

> She arrived at my office the following day at the appointed hour, marched in, and announced with some fanfare: "I am Ann." She promptly held up her car keys, dropped them on the floor, and sat down next to them with her dress carelessly draped about her. I asked if she would like to sit on a chair, stating that I would prefer that. She shook her head and looked at the rug. Then she raised her eyes, made a squinting grimace, and took her glasses off as if to show me her eyes. She shook her head from side to side in a rather stereotyped manner and exercised her jaw, but said nothing. (54)

This breach of the ritualized norms of therapy intensifies in subsequent sessions as Ann transgresses one of the fundamental boundaries of therapy: the line between the therapeutic and the personal. The interactions between Ann and her therapist in subsequent sessions are dominated by a struggle over this boundary:

> Our work in the beginning centered almost entirely on her demand that our relationship be something other than a professional one. She asked for special treatment and violated almost every conventional boundary that existed between us. For example, she would walk into my office swinging her arms so that I had to duck to avoid being hit in the head as she entered. From the start of treatment, she would call me at home at night following our sessions. During the therapy sessions, we struggled over innumerable parameters of treatment, such as whether or not she could lie on the analytic couch, whether she would have to sit in a chair or be allowed to sit on the floor and grab my legs, and whether or not she could call me at home between sessions. (58)

The therapist writes, "I did not feel her demands to be hostile but simply predatory: she wanted more of me" (59).

In addition to Ann's transgression of therapeutic boundaries, her psychiatric problems remain elusive to the therapist, as she refuses to provide the necessary material for the therapist to play his role. "She had no interest in giving me any information about the symptoms or problems that had brought her to psychiatric treatment in the first place. In fact, she seemed reluctant to be pinned down to any communication about specific complaints or to give any facts about her life. . . . My efforts to secure her history were met by Ann with smiles, grimaces, evasions, and non sequiturs" (55).

At the same time, Ann continues her scrutiny of her psychiatrist, attempting to extract from him information about his personal life. This attempt appears to him to be a defense against the therapy itself. "She said that she insisted on knowing all about me because she felt that, by being in psychotherapy, she was the one who was being treated as a specimen, 'like a butterfly pinned down by a collector to be scrutinized.' She felt that her only escape from such painful exploitation was to turn the tables on me and do to me what she feared psychotherapy was doing to her" (60).

Yet her psychiatrist refuses to provide the personal information she seeks, and this becomes a source of tension in the therapy. Demands for more information persist, and Ann's attempts at control within the therapy are accompanied by a dependence on the psychiatrist that intensifies in the course of the therapy.

Ann persists in her attempt to get information about her therapist, and at the same time, seems highly dependent on him. Her analyst states that she continually expressed the wish to be closer to him and even to be "one with him." She is extremely anxious during separations from him.

Ann's dependence on her therapist is illustrative of the increasing role of therapy in some women's lives, and their dependence on a paternalistic, benevolent helping profession, Ingleby's "psy complex." This dependence on the therapist as a parental figure or as a love object is a common theme in the borderline cases, as illustrated in this passage: "So powerful was her wish to be close to the analyst that she attempted to rent an apartment in the building where his office was located, an act which he learned of inadvertently from the building staff. . . . Her intense curiosity led her to try to find out all that she could about the analyst's personal life, and she continued at the same time to conceal her thoughts about him during her analytic sessions" (Abend 1983, 38).

Ann's transgression of the boundaries of their treatment relationship disrupts her psychiatrist's ability to work. When Ann is unexpectedly snowbound at the psychiatrist's house following a therapy session at his home office, he writes, "my own reaction to the evening was one of shock and dismay. I was confused about the effects that such an event would have on the treatment, and felt it likely that the work would be totally disrupted or hopelessly stymied by such a gross breach of the traditional boundaries of a therapeutic relationship" (Waldinger and Gunderson 1987, 63).

Ann's excessive neediness and "predatory" demands are translated into the language of pathology when the narrative shifts to the diagnosis of borderline personality disorder.

> Ann meets the DSM III criteria for Borderline Personality Disorder. At the start of this treatment she manifested inappropriate intense anger, identity disturbance, affective instability, intolerance of being alone, and chronic feelings of emptiness and boredom. She manifested little impulsivity and only mild self-destructiveness. In the sessions with her therapist, she clearly created an intense and unstable relationship. . . . Ann's psychological deficits at the start of treatment were considerable. Her childlike manner belied a striking capacity for regression to juvenile modes of functioning, as demonstrated by the immediacy with which she reverted to such behaviors in the therapist's office as grabbing his legs and refusing to sit in a chair. Moreover, she demonstrated considerable interpersonal boundary confusion, having difficulty differentiating her own thoughts and feelings from those of her therapist and of Dr. Brightman. (72)

As indicated in this passage, unpredictable behavior in the therapeutic situation is one important sign of borderline disorder. The analyst writes that Ann "created an intense and unstable relationship," a wording that makes Ann alone responsible for its intensity and instability. Ann's "juvenile" behavior in therapy is also mentioned as an important sign of her pathology.

Her therapist considers whether the diagnosis of hysteria—renamed "histrionic personality disorder" for the DSM-III—is appropriate for Ann:

The diagnosis of Histrionic Personality Disorder is suggested by Ann's overly dramatic, reactive, and intensely expressive behaviors. She was perceived by others as superficially charming but shallow. She lost function in ways that demanded that others take responsibility for her welfare and saw herself as a helpless person who needed constant reassurance. In fact, Ann fulfills the diagnostic criteria for Histrionic Personality Disorder. However, Ann's history of dissociative episodes, her devaluation of those who were important to her, her hostility, and her mild self-destructiveness are all more typical of a borderline disorder. (73)

Thus, while the hysteric is "overly dramatic," "charming but shallow," and helpless, all stereotypic feminine qualities; the borderline is more openly aggressive toward others and the self, suggesting the profile of the "demanding, aggressive, and angry woman" that Jimenez notes is the contemporary stereotyped image of the mentally disordered woman, the contemporary successor to the hysteric.

As these examples illustrate, some borderline patients appear to transgress the ritual boundaries of "normal" behavior in therapy. While on the one hand, such transgressions represent an intense dependence on, and demand of, their therapists, they also represent a refusal to play the role of "patient." Borderline patients are described as more actively demanding of the therapist as a person, rather than focusing on themselves.

This transgressive demand is, however, interpreted in psychiatric discourse as evidence of the patient's underlying borderline pathology—a pathological refusal to adhere to boundaries of normal social interaction, an oscillating and unstable identity. As a medical answer to the question of the patient's fluctuating behavior, the diagnosis of borderline becomes a sense-making device to manage the unpredictable patient. As Nathan Schwartz-Salant acknowledges, "A clinician's diagnosis of a patient as 'borderline' is often a kind of word magic, an apotropaic device to depotentiate and subdue this 'difficult patient'" (Schwartz-Salant 1989, 7).

A LANGUAGE OF LIQUIDS: RENDERING THE UNSTABLE FEMININE

Can it be that in the West, in our time, the female body has been constructed not only as a lack or absence but with more

complexity, as a leaking, uncontrollable, seeping liquid; as
formless flow; as viscosity, entrapping, secreting; as lacking not
so much or simply the phallus but self-containment—not a
cracked or porous vessel, like a leaking ship, but a formlessness
that engulfs all form, a disorder that threatens all order? (Grosz
1994, 203)

The rendering of the "unstable feminine" appears in more subtle
form in Melvin Singer's detailed study of borderline phenomenology in
an article in the *International Review of Psycho-Analysis* in 1977 (Singer
1977a; Singer 1977b). Appearing prior to the creation of the official
DSM definition in 1980, Singer's discussion delved into the nuances
of the self-experiences of the patients he deemed borderline. Though
not an individual case narrative (and hence not a chronological story
of a therapeutic encounter), Singer's account nonetheless provides many
descriptions of his analysands. Singer describes a pervasive symptom that
he finds in his borderline patients: "a chronic state of emptiness or being nothing, gone and missing," which can lead ultimately, Singer notes,
to the conviction of personal extinction (Singer 1977a, 460).

Metaphors constitute meaning through comparison or analogy, relying on given cultural codes or images. I would like to emphasize the
rhetorical construction of the borderline's unstable self through the
metaphor of liquidity or fluidity. Specifically, I examine how Singer
linguistically constructs the borderline patient's emptiness of self in the
narrative, projecting onto the borderline patient a literal intangibility
and fluidity of self that is culturally associated with femininity. Singer's
linguistic renderings of women diagnosed as borderline are highly
gendered, depicting the borderline's self or ego as intangible, fluid, misty,
ethereal—all culturally associated with the feminine. Women are defined in Singer's discourse negatively, as lacking the solid, firmly
bounded self.

The product of this narrative representation and interpretation is
a decontextual rendering of borderline subjectivity. While gender is explicitly excluded from the psychoanalytic interpretation offered in the
narrative (that is, the gendered context that makes the symptom meaningful), it nonetheless informs the linguistic representation of the borderline patient, reproducing gender stereotypes or cultural images of the
feminine.

Singer's discussion focuses on several female patients and one male patient who was experiencing gender and sexual conflicts. For such patients, this feeling of emptiness is frequently experienced as a physical feeling of hollowness or hunger; Singer notes that commonly heard symptoms include "hollowness, deadness, nothingness, an inner void, or 'something's missing'" (472). "Sudden or acute states of anguish and despair over this feeling of an inner world emptiness, especially when associated with an outer world emptiness (aloneness) are at times so exquisitely painful that suicide seems the only escape. Borderline patients dread the appearance of this emptiness and view it paradoxically as equivalent to a death experience—only a phenomenological, not physical death" (472).

Singer describes this experience as patients' loss of an "I," particularly in relation to powerful others. "Some borderline patients will describe a loss of their 'I' experience regardless of what it is, if the other person is too dominating—they fear getting swallowed up by the other's power. One patient, graphically and concretely, describes this loss of self in a dream, in which her face, although partially formed, was still without an 'eye'" (475).

Other cases describe the borderline patient's feelings of emptiness. In the case of Ginny, a borderline patient in private psychotherapy with Irvin Yalom, with whom she cowrote an account of their two years of therapy, she tells Dr. Yalom that her life is empty, speaking during one session, Yalom writes, of how "empty time was for her, beginning with the emptiness of writing in the morning which led into the emptiness of the rest of the day" (Yalom and Elkin 1974, 4). In Ginny's own narrative, she expresses an inability to define herself and a sense of detachment from both her surroundings and her self. She says that she "abandoned herself" long ago, and that this is why there is "no one there when I'm alone" (11). She uses the metaphor of a children's drawing board to describe her self: "When you lift up the paper," she writes," the easy funny faces, the squiggly lines, are all erased, leaving no traces" (xx).

Closely related to feelings of emptiness are feelings of numbness, or inner deadness, which are common themes in other clinical discussions. Richard Chessick notes that a pervasive symptom in his borderline patients is a feeling of being "alive but not alive" (Chessick 1977, 43). He discusses a case of a twenty-seven-year-old nun, who "felt continuously that she was dead. . . . She went through the motions of living always with a strange, almost indescribable feeling that she was not alive" (44). This did not cause concern, and she accepted it as her fate, notes Chessick, almost as if she had been born that way.

Chessick connects the experience of deadness to the need for physical touch. Chessick notes that the need for physical contact is so paramount in his borderline patients that they state that without this contact they do not feel alive. Chessick states that for these patients "some sort of profound sensation of deadness can only be neutralized by the physical touching presence of another human being and not by anything else" including "talk, psychotherapy, or interpretation of any kind" (45).

In another publication, Chessick presents the case of Trudy who suffers from "a deep sense of inner emptiness. There was a constant anguish about the meaninglessness of life and a perpetual feeling of boredom and indifference to everything. She had repeated fantasies of suicide, but made no attempts" (Chessick 1972, 769).

Singer describes his patients as cut off from object relations with others, relying on fragmentary feeling states or sensations to "anchor" their identities. According to Singer, his patients used these feeling states to ward off the horror of feelings of inner emptiness or deadness. For some patients, any physical feeling, whether pleasant or unpleasant, can become a kind of anchor point to the external world, providing a partial sliver of existence in place of a sense of internal void. "One borderline patient felt real, human, or some semblance of herself only when she experienced a queasy anxiety in the pit of her stomach which relieved her emptiness. This was her psychological center of gravity and she would look for that feeling to position herself in the world, to know who she was. Without anxiety, even if is was very discomforting, she felt as if she had disappeared or was nothing" (Singer 1977b, 473).

Aside from such physical anchor points to ward off the threat of extinction of self, Singer notes another, perhaps more disturbing strategy of being in the face of nothingness, where the patient constructs a nonhuman, or even inanimate "false self." Some patients create fantasied, nonhuman selves, thereby turning themselves into objects: "In this way, they had defensively already died, so they could not be abandoned and thus suffer the excruciating agony of annihilation of the self." To preserve their fragmentary and fleeting selves, Singer's women patients construct a state of "living death" to survive in a kind of subdued state, neither fully alive nor dead, at the border. They feel like objects, or parts of the scenery: like a "blade of grass" or "like the scenery": "One woman, in the secrecy of her inner thoughts, felt she must be like a tree, since she did not feel human. She knew that her parents were human, but since they did not attend to her, she felt she was more like the scenery, which is also unattended. Thus, she might as well be a tree which at least has roots deep in the ground" (474).

These descriptions present a language of the borderline self as fluid, intangible, dissoluble. Singer's language is revealing of the metaphoric connotations he has layered onto the borderline's sense of inner emptiness. The narrative invokes the cultural signifiers of abjection, in its representation of the non-self of the borderline as permeable and shifting, and Singer notes that his patients themselves appear to have a horror of the lack of solidity.

Singer describes the borderline patient's defensive false part-selves as their attempts to combat the "dissolution" or fluidity of the empty self. Masochism, for example, is described as a way for patients to avoid dissolving:

> Another common method used by borderline patients to
> preserve this self-experience and to feel alive is to suffer
> masochistically, be excited, or in danger. Thus, by bombarding
> the outer boundaries of the body or psychic self with painful
> stimuli, cathexis is kept at the periphery and a sense of intact-
> ness, definition, delineation and aliveness is temporarily
> achieved. Hardness, physical pain and psychic combativeness
> gives some borderline patients the feeling of definition and
> limits, not unbounded extensiveness and dissolution. (474)

Such descriptive terms as "hardness" and "intactness" express Singer's notion of the flip side of the empty, fluid, dissolved self—one characterized by solidity, firmness, and constancy over time. But such "hard" defenses don't always hold the fluid self inside its borders: "I have treated two patients who described feeling like a block of ice. The difficulty with this defensive posture is that one can readily be melted with the heat of emotions and become nothing but a puddle of water" (474).

Singer also describes a type of borderline patient who keeps up a continual flow of talk, which he interprets as a wish to merge with the analyst by maintaining constant contact with him, and to avoid a sense of separateness. Such a flow of talk, which Singer likens to the need for "small talk," is accompanied by "inexorable panic when the person feels any degree of 'me' feelings separate from 'us.'" Again, a liquid metaphor is invoked here as Singer describes incessant talk as "equivalent to feeding and a continual flow of milk and urine" (474).

In addition to using metaphors of liquidity, Singer describes the intangibility of the empty self as mist or smoke: "Other patients used the reverse defense to avoid dissolution: rather than hard firmness, they present a misty, airy smoke-screen effect which dynamically expresses their lack of structural integrity while simultaneously keeping the other away, unpenetrating and safely uninvolved" (474).

In another example, Singer depicts the dissolution of self in highly gendered terms, counterposing a feminine "dissolution" with masculine intactness:

> One woman, mentioned above, feared closeness, especially
> close physical contact, with another woman not primarily
> because of homosexual danger, although that certainly was
> present, but on this same level, out of her fear of dissolution
> into the other woman. She chose hard, muscular men whose
> firmness made her feel insoluble: into whom she could press but
> not sink and fall, dispersed into an eternally bottomless abyss.
> Her desire, it seemed, was to press into the other's body—
> through the outer integument, and insinuate herself between
> the muscles, tendons and fasciae. Here the merger, closeness
> and warmth of the other's body, especially the outer rind, was
> primary. (477)

The use of metaphors of liquidity to refer to women reproduces the cultural association of femininity with the material "flows" of nature. Klaus Theweleit, in his analysis of the writings of Freikorps soldiers in prefascist Germany, found that floods and flows were central metaphors used to represent the threat of the emergent socialist revolution, the Red Tide that threatened Germany from within its borders, and that this flood was equated with the threat of women. Women became a "code word for the whole complex of nature" in the writings of the

Freikorps soldiers (Theweleit 1987, 215). The image of "woman-in-the-water" is one running through Western literature, "over and over again: the women-in-the-water; woman as water, as a stormy, cavorting, cooling ocean, a raging stream, a waterfall; as a limitless body of water that ships pass through, with tributaries, pools, surfs, and deltas; woman as the enticing (or perilous) deep." This imagery is a "depersonalization of women . . . the dissolving of their boundaries" (283). "What is really at work here, it seems to me, is a specific (and historically relatively recent) form of the oppression of women—one that has been notably underrated. It is oppression through exaltation, through a lifting of boundaries, an 'irrealization' and reduction to principle—the principle of flowing, of distance, of vague, endless enticement. Here again, women have no names" (284).

Theweleit explores the relationship of these metaphors to the anxiety of the Freikorps "soldier males" over the dissolution of their own boundaries, particularly those of male identity, of the body, and of the "pure" race of Germany: "Our soldiers, conversely, want to avoid swimming at all costs, no matter what the stream. They want to stand with both feet and every root firmly anchored in the soil. They want whatever floods may come to rebound against them; they want to stop, and dam up, those floods" (230).

Singer reads a diverse array of women's symptoms as signs of the literal intangibility and solubility of the borderline's empty self. For Singer, these experiences are signs of an underlying structural flaw in the patient's self. He interprets the borderline symptoms as defenses against facing the horror of this emptiness and dissolution. Thus, for Singer, the borderline patients' selves are indeed dissolved, fluid, insubstantial—and this lack of a stable self causes mental anguish.

We might read Singer's language as unconsciously signifying a cultural disquiet about the permeability of borders of the clean, demarcated body or self. As Grosz writes, "What is disturbing about the viscous or the fluid is its refusal to conform to the laws governing the clean and proper, the solid and the self-identical, its otherness to the notion of an entity—the very notion that governs our self-representations and understanding of the body" (Grosz 1994, 195).

Singer notes that borderline patients are especially vulnerable to the strains of the psychoanalytic situation, due to their tenuous and intangible self-experience. Here, too, Singer brings diverse behaviors, including responses to the strains peculiar to the analytic situation, under the umbrella of the dissolved emptiness of borderline patients. Singer notes that borderline patients' vulnerability to the psychoanalytic situation "attest[s] to the remarkable instability and flimsy quality of the borderline's defensive self-experience." (Singer 1977b, 475). Yet an alternative reading of these responses by borderline patients suggests that they are responding to the power differentials of the psychoanalytic situation itself. For example, some patients "feared unlimited and unbounded free association," for it "opens them up to infinity and psychological annihilation, since they cannot grasp or get hold of any continuity and coherence of their thought, and thus of themselves" (475). Another patient "said she felt she had to [be] silent, for she feared—quite irrationally, she realized—that if I listened to her, how she felt, thought, etc., then she was in my mind not hers, and she would be nothing. Her silence kept her belonging to herself" (475).

Another patient was afraid to reveal cherished stories from childhood: "These tales were the very fabric of her partial sense of worth and completeness as a person—all she had, to fill, in any gratifying way, the void in her inner life as well as provide a sense of self, i.e., 'I am this person with this wretched history'" (476).

Silence as a strategy of control in a situation of power is not necessarily without rationality. The "fundamental rule" of psychoanalysis—free association—is that the patient should say anything and everything, without censoring it. Yet psychoanalysis itself is based on the analysts' silence, and breaks a fundamental rule of everyday speech, as Clément points out, to provide an answer: "Not answering, breaking the circuit of normal communication—that's the brilliant, fundamental trick of Freud's practice" (Clément 1987, 78). This silence itself is meant to encourage the free flow of speech: "On this paradox—on the patient's quickness to overfill the emotional vacuum created by the analyst's reticence—the analysis is poised, and it may as easily founder as take off" (Malcolm 1982, 38). Yet, as Foucault has shown, the silence of the analyst is the power and privilege of a listener who does not share in the obligation to speak, and the obligation to speak is itself not necessarily the liberation of "truth" from the individual, but is akin to a mode of confession, which reaches its completion in the silent listener who judges (Foucault 1980).

Yet for Singer, this fear is irrational and a sign of "pathology," not only of a "general disturbance of self, but of a generalized state of 'undifferentiatedness'" (Singer 1977b, 475). Borderline patients' "holding on" to their stories is portrayed in relation to unconscious preservation of inner bodily contents or fluids: "Borderline patients, in this state of regressed cognitive-perceptual, primary process functioning and drive orientation, conceive of everything in narcissistic oral-anal terms, as inside or outside, retaining or expelling bodily contents" (475).

Singer juxtaposes this fear of analytic power with another symptomatic fear, that of "falling in love": "One woman feared falling in love, for then she would give all of herself to the other and be left with nothing" (475).

Building on his assumption that patients' feelings of depersonalization and deadness are in actuality strategies for avoiding the horror of inner emptiness, Singer is able to interpret a wide variety of symptoms as additional signs of the borderline patient's underlying intangibility and fluidity. This occurs when Singer shifts his attention from emptiness to other symptoms or behaviors that are viewed as strategies used to avoid the empty self.

For example, while the patient for whom queasy anxiety in the pit of her stomach wards off feelings of nonexistence is viewed as avoiding the horror of emptiness, so too there are a variety of other behaviors in which the connection to an actual underlying emptiness appears more tenuous. In the following statement regarding that patient, who "lived every feeling to its completion, be it hunger, anger, or sex," Singer links a variety of characteristics to this single underlying cause:

> This revelation, during the course of her modified psychoanaly-
> sis—i.e. that she linked keeping alive her feelings to her
> aliveness as a person—was a major determinant in helping to
> curb her promiscuity. It eventually led to her increasing ability
> to tolerate more frustration, which through further insight and
> integration led to the development of a more cohesive sense of
> self. This preoccupation with aliveness to avoid emptiness, in
> this same individual, was also responsible for her insistence on

being constantly active not passive. Passively watching TV sent her into a panic. . . . Likewise, maintaining this "alive" self was one of the bases for her self-centredness, rigid control and exhibitionism. (473)

Singer is speaking here about a variety of behaviors and reactions: promiscuity, intolerance of frustration, self-centeredness, exhibitionism. While details about the patient are not provided here, it is evident from this description that Singer believes her to be too self-present, promiscuous, demanding, and controlling. It could equally be argued that this patient was striving for mastery and control over her own selfhood in her life and in the analytic situation itself. Yet these strivings are, for Singer, ultimately "false"—not part of the self.

Singer ties these diverse responses and conflicts to the literal intangibility and solubility of the borderline's empty self. What are excluded from the presentation are any details about the context of his patients' lives, their social situation, or even their personal histories. Signs of the dissolved empty self are presented in an isolated, decontextualized fashion, in the form of a listing of examples. Given that his concern is with this decontextualized symptom as signs of the empty self, he forgoes discussion of the connection between borderline patients' experiences of emptiness and numbness to gender conflicts.

I am not suggesting that Singer consciously or intentionally portrays his borderline patients as lacking or negatively defined. Rather, I am interested in the implications of the metaphor of emptiness as an organizing scheme in the narrative, and how it becomes a defining feature of depictions of the borderline patient's unstable self. Singer builds his narrative around this metaphor, and thus from the borderline patient's expressed sense of emptiness, Singer infers a deep structure that has gone awry or dissolved. Other analysts, too, shift from statements about what the patient is expressing about her experience of emptiness to statements about the patient as actually empty. As Chessick states, in the early stages of Trudy's therapy, "I felt I was dealing with a character disorder or borderline patient, who was very empty and in a chaotic state" (Chessick 1972, 769). Yalom, too, is preoccupied with Ginny's empty state, writing, "She is drawn to emptiness like a magnet and sucks it up and spits it out in front of me. One would think that nothing in her life existed except nothingness" (Yalom and Elkin 1974, 4).

EMPTINESS AND THE "BAD MOTHER"

Singer offers a fuller psychoanalytic interpretation of the roots of the borderline's emptiness and intangibility that finally seals the boundary between a concern for an inner void and a more contextualized gendered understanding. Singer writes that emptiness can be understood as the patient's internalization of a fantasied "bad mother." Singer draws upon Melanie Klein's notion of infant development, which postulates that aggression is as powerful a drive as libido at birth, and that infants project both aggressive and libidinal fantasies onto their mothers. The infant's image of the mother, therefore, is split into a fantasied "good mother" and an evil "bad mother." Infants then reinternalize, or "introject," these images of the mother as inner object representations, which make up part of the self. As Singer states, "borderline emptiness can be portrayed, in part, as an agonizing self-image of being nothing, based on the introjection and primary identification with the mother who is equally empty" (Singer 1977b, 478).

Singer offers a case example of a woman whose dreams were plagued by images of "malevolent male intruders" who invaded her bedroom at night in the form of ghosts. For Singer, these "ghosts" represent external images of emptiness that the patient has projected onto the world. Singer notes that the etymological root of the word "ghost" is Germanic and means "fury." In mythology, ghosts can "at one and the same time be hollow or empty and yet full of evil." The archaic psychic evil that has been internalized as a bad inner object representation of the mother can be projected onto the world again, in the form of ghosts:

> One female patient experienced herself at different times as different "selves." On some occasions of elevated self-esteem she felt like a successful career woman. This self-image was related to the self-esteem of powerful phallic masculine identifications. At other times she felt and looked like a little latency girl bedecked with pigtails, pranks and brattiness. However, her truly pathognomonic self-image was the empty self which she depicted with utter horror. At such times she would describe her body interior as totally hollow, empty. . . . She would dream of malevolent male intruders whom she chased from her bedroom, but who escaped through the cracks in her window-sills by turning into non-corporeal beings. Associations led to the frequent "disappearance" and

abandonment by her mother and then to her own childhood
fear of ghosts and of being alone in the night. Further associations brought to light memories in which she thought of herself
alone on a mountain top, screaming for help—but the only
response was her own hollow, companion-like echo. This stark,
barren empty, lonely state was a reflexion of her utterly unbearable feeling of emptiness and these ghost-like, evanescent,
shadowy invaders seemed to represent external representations
of her own empty, internalized, greedy and devouring self- and
object introjects. (478)

What might this story suggest, aside from emptiness? The reference
to a scattered, vacillating self-image split between the "little latency girl"
and a "successful career woman" suggests the ambivalent, divided views
of the culture toward women—adult women being haunted by an image of dependency and childishness that subverts their efforts at empowerment. And empowerment, here, can come only in the form of
"phallic masculine identifications." With no power of her own, and with
an "empty" or evil mother image haunting her imagination of self,
Singer's narrative suggests, the borderline patient is condemned to only
fleeting identities. This example is revealing of the limited binary op-
tions between masculine identification and feminine passivity. The only
option between masquerading as a man and posing as a "little latency
girl" is the void of borderline subjectivity: the empty self.

Object relations analysts interpret borderline symptoms as aberrations in the normal course of the construction of a self. The assumption at work in the narratives is that if the self is given the proper
maternal narcissistic mirroring, it will have the means by which to un-
fold, internalizing the qualities of the mother in forming an integrated,
balanced, and stable sense of self. In this account, the surrounding culture is not problematized as a set of conditions within which persons
acquire senses of self.

Male Borderlines: Emotional Rigidity and
the Hypervigilant Self

When men are diagnosed as borderline, how is their self pathology
described? How are such descriptions related to gender discourse? Spe-

cifically, how is the theme of instability depicted in case narratives of men?

The case of Stewart, the only male case in the series of cases discussed by Waldinger and Gunderson (1987), illustrates some of the different ways male borderlines are described and interpreted. Stewart is a twenty-year-old who has been hospitalized for suicidal impulses and "intrusive and bizarre thoughts that had recurred over the preceding several months" (80). These include images of his dead cousin's body and fears that he is being somehow influenced and followed by staff at a local business establishment.

Stewart's narrative features many of the same themes as the cases of women. One prominent theme is Stewart's resistance to therapy. For example, one of the main conflicts in the analysis revolves around Stewart's reluctance to give a narrative to his analyst and his suspicion of the analyst regarding his motives. He also violates the norms of therapy, and begins smoking and eating during his sessions. There are numerous conflicts over payment of his bill for therapy. He tends to berate the hospital staff and his parents, and he refuses to cooperate in family therapy with his parents.

Stewart's resistance takes the form of intense anger directed toward his analyst:

> After my return from vacation, Stewart entered the most
> intense and unremitting period of rage in his therapy. The
> subjects of this rage were my failure to provide him with what
> he needed and my having "addicted him to therapy," taking all
> of his money so that he could have no pleasures in his life. He
> acted out about paying bills and about arriving at and leaving
> sessions at times designated by me. I spent a great deal of time
> interpreting these maneuvers as his efforts to regain a sense of
> control over me and as reactions to his recognition that I could
> and would let him leave. He acknowledged the former but
> angrily denied the latter. He spent therapy hours in angry
> tirades about these subjects, followed by periods of silence and a
> contemptuous and overtly sadistic attitude that made it difficult
> for me to maintain my equanimity. (89)

The conflicts between Stewart and his analyst coalesce in Stewart's rage when his analyst raises the issue of termination of therapy. "He complained that I had created a need in him" (89).

Yet Stewart's borderline self pathology is described differently than that of female borderline patients. One important feature is lacking in descriptions of Stewart: instability, particularly of emotions, but also of self. The authors write that he presented a "less classical picture of Borderline Personality Disorder than others in our group (e.g. Susan, Martha)." Rather than an unstable, fluid, ever-changing self, he appears to have a rigid, controlled personality: "Certainly, he did not present with the hungry, needy quality that many borderline patients exhibit. His superficial coldness and aloof style, his guarded demeanor, and his intolerance of the wishes of others are characteristic of the narcissistic personality" (99).

He also has the characteristics of another diagnosis more frequently given to men, paranoid personality disorder. "Stewart exhibited pervasive, unwarranted mistrust of people—most notably his therapist. He was guarded and hypervigilant, and was constantly suspicious of other's motives" (99).

Further, even though Stewart expresses "inappropriate intense anger, violent impulses"—about which the authors note, he was "the only member of our group who reported significant violent impulses that were sometimes acted upon (damage to property)"—as well as "impulsivity and self-damaging acts," these emotions and actions were not interpreted as signs of instability. The analysts conclude that "he did not demonstrate significant affective instability" (99). Thus, unlike in the cases of women, Stewart's rage was not viewed as evidence of an unstable self.

It may be that this is an instance of men's anger not being pathologized in the way that women's is. Joan Busfield attributes this perception to the tendency to view men as more rational. "Men . . . are constituted as more independent, tough-minded and rational, and when they display the emotions of rage and hate, this is less likely to be constituted as being 'emotional'" (Busfield 1996, 107).

This perception becomes all the more interesting in light of Stewart's revealing that he read extensively on Hitler, "whom he admired and envied for his enormous powers" (86). He had childhood fantasies of being a "victorious military conqueror," which he remembered having when he felt very "small" in the face of his father's temper and his sister's teasing (87). He comes to realize that he felt comfortable being angry at others and didn't want attachments to anyone. "All I am is angry," he states. "I need people to hate" (93).

His analyst interprets his hostility as a defensive adaptation to his insecurity in relationships with others. Rather than being excessively needy, Stewart actively denies having needs. "He found his own dependency needs intolerable, and so assumed a counter-dependent stance that alienated others. . . . He routinely withdrew from the threats and frustrations of interpersonal relationships into schizoid fantasies of a grandiose nature. This withdrawal and grandiosity were accompanied by harsh devaluation of others" (100).

The picture that emerges of Stewart is one of a rigid personality that is hostile and defensive. The focus of the narrative is on the outer defensive and paranoid expressions in his relations with others and with the analyst, and does not discuss in detail the underlying instability of self. In the commentary on the case the authors note that "the therapist did not conceive of Stewart's behavioral disturbances as based on ego deficits, but rather held that the patient was capable of more responsible behavior and had to take responsibility for his refusal to utilize that capability" (102).

The themes of defensive personality and rigid control are prominent in another male case, "Dr. X," appearing, like the case of Stewart, in a monograph of several cases in which he is the only male (Abend et al. 1983). Dr. X is introduced to the reader as a "twenty-three-year-old single Jewish medical student when he began his ten year analysis" (50). Born during World War II, the patient was in therapy during the 1970s. He enters therapy because he is failing medical school and is depressed about his parents' divorce. He has also begun to fight with his mother, who he feels is overprotective of him. He both fears and admires his father, who is also a physician whom Dr. X describes as "insensitive, mocking, impatient, and sarcastic" (54).

Dr. X's feelings toward his parents are mirrored in his relationships with women and men. His narrative is characterized by the themes of avoidance of women and fear of, rivalry, and competition with other men. He avoids long-term relationships with women, fearing they are trying to tie him down and trap him. "He once said that he feared that a woman 'would suck me up into her as though she were a vacuum cleaner'" (55). In addition, his analyst writes that "he consciously thought that his mother might want to sexually seduce him" (55). These beliefs, his analyst writes, are "persistent and severe and he had many quasiparanoid feelings," thus placing him close to the borderline of psychosis.

He feels that men, including the analyst, might "prove him wrong and thus humiliate him" (56). His fears of humiliation by men intensify in the transference when he suspects that the analyst wants him to "give in" by showing emotion. "He was convinced that the analyst had ulterior motives to ensnare him and humiliate him. He felt that the analyst would force him to give in—to admit his childish needs or to admit that the analyst was correct and he was wrong. Then his analyst would have overpowered him and made him weak, small and stupid" (59).

While Dr. X, like Stewart and other borderline patients, is described as being resistant in therapy, his resistance is even more veiled and indirect. "Unlike those transference reactions of borderline patients which are stormy, impulsive, and dramatic in their intensity, this patient's transference feelings were hidden and silent. He acted as though he was wary and mistrustful of the analyst and the treatment, although he denied having such feelings. He said rather early on, when the analyst made some attempt at understanding his transference feelings, that he was not going to have *any* feelings toward the analyst" (54).

As the narrative progresses, a crucial incident from the patient's past emerges: His mother had an infant girl who died after birth, causing the mother to become severely depressed. This incident becomes the backdrop for the description of several fantasies and dreams involving either cross-gender or homosexual themes. In one fantasy, Dr. X is with a seductive older woman, who demands that he become a little girl. He reports having a dream during a period when he wasn't seeing the analyst, that the analyst is performing a sexual act on him. "He thought to himself 'So that is why he is treating me!' . . . He was shocked by this dream because it made him wonder whether his suspicions about the analyst doing something to him had anything to do with this fantasy" (58). He reveals that at age thirteen he would put on his mother's underwear and dresses and look into the mirror. He expresses much shame about these fantasies.

The analyst explains why Dr. X is diagnosed as borderline:

> This patient was considered to be borderline because of the pervasiveness of the psychopathology, which involved almost every area of his functioning. . . . His pathology invaded his entire character structure and was of a relatively stable degree with no severe regression to psychosis. His reality testing was impaired, especially in the areas of his object relations, where he viewed women as trapping and ensnaring him. He also, for many years, thought his mother might actually wish to seduce him. His object relations were also characterized by marked suspicion and mistrust. He had few friends and always felt he would be humiliated or scorned by men. (62–63)

Like Stewart, Dr. X is depicted not as emotionally unstable, but as emotionally "overcontrolled" and rigid. This is expressed in the transference:

> In contrast to other borderline patients whose transference reactions are characterized as immediately intense, impulsive, excessively clinging, or openly hostile, this patient's transference was revealed in, and hidden by, a rigid, unfeeling, unemotional facade. The defensive quality of this behavior became clear in the course of treatment. . . . His affects were overcontrolled, leading to an appearance of rigidity of his personality. There was a marked inability to accept the "as if" quality of the transference. He tried to elicit countertransference feelings of helplessness, defeat, and humiliation in the analyst of the sort which had marked his own suffering as a child. (63)

The cases of Stewart and Dr. X thus depict a form of rigid, controlled, unemotional personality, a hypervigilance that might be said to reflect a kind of exaggerated depiction of hegemonic masculinity. These two cases contrast with the women's cases, in depicting the borderline disorder in men not as instability, but as a kind of hypercontrol, lack of emotion, and overly rigid personality style.

However, in each of these cases, the theme of homosexuality is hinted at as an underlying trend that threatens to destabilize the patient's rigid control (or that provides a partial explanation of destabilization). This theme is even more prominent in other cases, which provide evidence of Joel Paris's comment that men who receive the diagnosis of borderline are homosexual. In these cases, in contrast to the depiction of an exaggerated masculinity expressed in the cases of Stewart and Dr. X, men's borderline "pathology" is interpreted in relation to failures or lapses in masculinity. Gender and sexuality confusion figures prominently in the constellation of identity conflicts associated with borderline disorder in men. Melvin Singer, for example, mentions only one male patient, and in particular writes of this patient's conflicts with homosexuality and feminine gender identification:

> When one male patient realized, in revelatory fashion, that he had a fantasy of being a female homosexual (which was a partial basis for his anxiety over sexual contact with women since that meant that he was not just, as he thought, a male homosexual, but actually a female homosexual) rather than experience relief from some of his distress and greater social freedom during the working through process, he became, for period of time, more anxious, withdrawn, and despondent. But now, not because of homosexual acting out [here homosexuality is defined as deviance] but because of increased emptiness and anxiety with the threat of non-existence from giving up this homosexual fantasy to the integrative work of his conscious rational mind. I had taken away the only part of his personality that had any substance, value or that he knew of, or sensed, if only in a slight way. He felt now, "more like an empty shell." (Singer 1977b, 476)

Similarly, in "The Borderline Diathesis," Manuel Ross discusses one female patient and one male patient, in the context of theoretical comments about the borderline's "central defect . . . in the organizing structures of the self" (Ross 1976, 308). Ross defines the central defect of the borderline patient as the absence or defectiveness of the "organizing forms of the self which give life its richness and a certain dimension" (309). Each of Ross's patients behaves in ways that contradict gender expectations. Agnes is aggressive and expresses rage directed at Ross. Carl, like the patient in Singer's example, experiences sexual and gender identity conflicts: "In his first hour, he wanted to know if I could tell him whether he was homosexual or not" (318). Carl's family background includes a father who was physically abusive to his wife and children, and a mother who was "seductive and infantalizing" with Carl. His father "had bragged of being a tough and had tried to spin around himself a picture of masculinity" (318). Carl was teased by his peers as being a "mama's boy," "but for the most part he denied it and the problems of separation through an identification with the father's pseudo-masculinity" (318). Ross then states, "The deeper unconscious identification was with his mother along the lines of 'I need never lose my mother. I've become a woman like her.' Yet, he yearned for an identification with a strong man other than the identification with the aggressor that had taken place with his father" (318). Ross relates an anonymous homosexual encounter Carl experienced in a men's bathroom stall when he was thirteen, and also describes Carl's failed attempt to become a marine. Initially, Carl was hopeful that this would affirm his masculinity: "He was sure, at least, that he had at last taken that decisive step towards 'becoming a man'" (319). However, the abusive treatment he received from the drill sergeant made him wish to escape, and he confessed his homosexuality to the camp psychiatrist, and was discharged.

These cases of men diagnosed as borderline show that the male borderline's self is depicted not as unstable, but as rigid, defensive, and hypervigilant, a stance that resembles culturally defined standards of masculinity. Thus, masculinity here does not escape pathologization. As Joan Busfield points out, "The 'acting out' of masculinity, most obviously through certain forms of sexual and physical violence, can be deemed evidence of mental disturbance as the categories of criminal insanity and psychopathy attest, and there are male images of mental disorder no less than female" (Busfield 1996, 104). Yet she emphasizes that men tend to be perceived as antisocial and are controlled through the criminal justice system, rather than being deemed mad. Yet those men such as Carl, who show lapses in culturally defined masculinity, are viewed as unstable, suggesting that selfhood and gender display are inextricably linked in the perception of the "normal" self.

Conclusion

The detailed narratives of those abject women deemed borderline provide a rich landscape in which to examine the contradictions of gender subjectivity and how it is represented. This chapter demonstrates the complexities of women's relation to selfhood and subjectivity—through an examination of the psychoanalytic and psychotherapeutic case narratives of women whose selves are deemed unstable. With feminist analyses of the position of Woman as Other, in the interstices or borderlines of culture, as a backdrop, I have explored the connections between these cultural meanings of femininity and the depictions of feminine self-pathology in psychoanalytic discourse.

The narratives depict this cultural and symbolic marginality with reference to the patients' outward appearance, which is said to be "off-center," as Stein noted. The borderline patient is also described as particularly unpredictable or incomprehensible. Ann, for example, resists conforming to the norms and rituals of therapy, and transgresses the boundaries between patient and analyst, with her "predatory" demands on her therapist. Analysts also focus on the patient's outward appearance as a sign of an inner disturbance or incoherence of self, as illustrated in Stein's discussion of Ms. V., who displays an exaggerated, monstrous feminine appearance that he describes as "off-center."

These textual depictions of the borderline patient can be viewed as psychoanalysts' attempts to make sense of the borderline patient's unpredictable behavior, and of her "uncanny" qualities. Analysts have strong transferential relations to the borderline patient, and their formal psychiatric or psychoanalytic interpretations of these patients must be viewed in this light. The situational context of therapy, frequently becoming a struggle between patient and analyst (as in the case of Ann) or a tension or silence, with an "uncanny" quality, is not a neutral medium for interpretation of the patient.

The formal interpretation of the patient from the object relations framework, which defines the self as a gender-neutral, coherent, and bounded entity, yields an ahistorical and decontextualized reading of the borderline patient's symptoms as an inner pathology. Further, the source of this pathology is frequently traced to the mother, an interpretation that serves to elide the context of the patriarchal culture within which women construct selves.

In addition to this formal interpretation using psychoanalytic theory, there is the linguistic construction of the unstable borderline self. Singer, for example, vividly reconstructs his borderline patient's "tenuous self-experience," relying on the metaphors of emptiness and liquidity to depict the borderline patient's self as dissolving, fluid, and intangible.

Overall, this analysis of the cases shows the way in which women diagnosed as borderline are perceived as not fitting into the norm of the "self": Their selves are plural, not unitary; incoherent or split, not integrated and coherent; empty, not full; dissolving and vacillating, not with firm borders. Women diagnosed as borderline appear to their analysts to be without firm self borders—as in the analysis of Ginny, who exhibits a "strange diffuseness, a blurring of ego boundaries," and as in Singer's patients, whose selves, Singer theorizes, are at risk of dissolving. The more infrequent cases of men diagnosed borderline, by contrast, are described as rigid and defensive, and their rage is not defined as evidence of an emotionally or structurally unstable self. Yet lapses in masculinity, signaled by a so-called deviant sexual orientation and what are perceived as more feminine behaviors, are linked in the narratives with the threat of destabilization of self. Coherent and stable selfhood, then, in these analysts' view, depends upon culturally condoned expressions of gender.

Chapter 4	Fragmented Selves

Borderline Case Narratives

CHAPTER 3 ANALYZED the linguistic depiction of women diagnosed as borderline in the case narratives, focusing on the narrative construction of borderline women as fluid, unstable, and lacking a coherent, unified self. This chapter explores one particular manifestation of instability discussed in the case narratives: the theme of fragmentation or splitting of selfhood. Singer understands his patients as having constructed various "false selves" to cover over and bind the underlying emptiness and dissolution of self, thus leaving them with split or fragmented selves. In the cases discussed here, the theme of split selfhood is even more pronounced. The borderline patient's instability is described as arising from a self that is split or fragmented between a false, surface self or "mask"; and an inner realm of either emptiness, as in Singer's patients, or repressed or buried parts of the self that do not or cannot find expression in the patient's outward behavior. These patients are thus left with unintegrated selves, oscillating between an artificial surface conformity and an abject emptiness. Here I focus in more detail on this theme of fragmented or split selfhood in several case narratives, examining how this fragmentation is depicted and interpreted.

This analysis explores the potential for a feminist cultural reading of the fragmentation of self expressed by women and recounted in the case narratives. I seek to situate such fragmented selfhood in the gendered and cultural context within which women construct subjectivity, in order to analyze the construction of "false selves" as a response to contradictory cultural meanings of femininity.

Elaine Showalter points out that in the period after 1930, hysteria was no longer the predominant female diagnosis, having been eclipsed by another diagnosis widely applied to women: schizophrenia. Schizophrenia is a psychotic disorder, marked by auditory or visual hallucinations and disorganized thought processes. However, during the 1950s it was defined more broadly and applied more loosely, particularly for women. In Carol Warren's analysis of women in the 1950s who had been hospitalized for schizophrenia, a reanalysis of the case histories of women revealed that only half could be confidently diagnosed as schizophrenic; the other half either were "definitely not" schizophrenic, or their status was "uncertain" (Warren 1987, 26–27). Such uncertain cases, close as they are to the border of psychosis, today might very well have met a definition of borderline disorder.

Showalter offers a feminist analysis of this modern female malady. "Schizophrenic symptoms of passivity, depersonalization, disembodiment, and fragmentation have parallels in the social situation of women" (Showalter 1985, 213). What is most relevant for the analysis of borderline narratives is the conception of a female subjectivity split between outward appearance of the body as object, and inner subjecthood. Examining the autobiographical narratives of female asylum patients, she notes that schizophrenic women have the sense of themselves as "unoccupied bodies. Feeling that they have no secure identities, the women look to external appearances for confirmation that they exist. Thus they continually look at their faces in the mirror, but out of desperation rather than narcissism" (212). Showalter interprets this split as an exaggeration of women's "normal" state, citing John Berger's comment that women have a double role as actor and spectator, as surveyor and surveyed. "A woman must continually watch herself. She is almost continually accompanied by her own image of herself. . . . From earliest childhood she has been taught and persuaded to survey herself continually. And so she comes to consider the surveyor and surveyed within her as the two constituent yet always distinct elements of her identity as a woman" (Berger, cited in Showalter 1985,

212). As Showalter notes, "Some feminist critics have maintained that schizophrenia is the perfect literary metaphor for the female condition, expressive of women's lack of confidence, dependency on external, often masculine, definitions of the self, split between the body as sexual object and the mind as subject, and vulnerability to conflicting social messages about femininity and maturity" (212).

Showalter sees poet Sylvia Plath's autobiographical fiction *The Bell Jar* as expressing in complex ways these conflicts and splits, and notes that the heroine in the novel, Esther, is "split between the feminine and the creative selves" (217). Esther believes that "Motherhood and writing . . . are incompatible. Esther's sense of an absolute division between her creativity and her femininity is the basis of her schizophrenia" (216). Fearing being trapped by motherhood and marriage in a life she doesn't want, and facing scorn or denial of her writing, as well as a sense that women who do have "careers" are denied love, Esther faces a double bind in which she must choose between two mutually opposed and seemingly separate existences. This impasse is poignantly illustrated in Esther's vision of her future as a fig tree with a series of futures represented by the figs on the branches, one representing a "husband and a happy home and children." Others represent illustrious writing careers—a "famous poet," a "brilliant professor"; or "Ee Gee, the amazing editor." Another fig is a series of lovers. Esther sees that she cannot choose more than one, since under the societal constraints of female identity "choosing one meant losing all the rest, and as I sat there, unable to decide, the figs began to wrinkle and go black, and, one by one, they plopped to the ground at my feet" (Plath 1971, 63).

Caught in the impasse, Esther is unable to imagine a future, and feels "very still and very empty, the way the eye of a tornado must feel" (2). Showalter's analysis suggests that Esther's madness is a meaningful response to irreconcilable and mutually exclusive images for women's identity, a split that Esther embodies in her oscillations between writing and love, and in her paralysis, depression, and emptiness.

My analysis draws on Showalter's analysis of madness as an exaggeration of the cultural double binds of feminine identity to analyze the fragmented self depicted in the borderline narratives.

Masks of Femininity: Ms. V.

In a clinical article published in 1929, "Womanliness as Masquerade," Joan Riviere describes the behavior of some of her women patients as a "masquerade" of femininity, the putting on of an exaggerated mask of feminine traits, in order to disguise or cover a fantasized forbidden "masculine" self. Riviere suggests that her patients are divided into a strategically performed artificial femininity and some forbidden aspect of self that, when exposed or performed, is threatening to others, and makes her the target of retribution. Riviere traces this fantasy to a desire to take the position of men, and more specifically, to a rivalry with the father in an oedipal drama (Riviere 1929).

The themes of artificiality and superficiality are frequently seen in the borderline case narratives. The patient is said to express feelings of artificiality or falsity, which often accompany sensations of emptiness and numbness. This is described as a superficial, surface mask or persona that is a kind of empty adaptation to the surroundings.

For Yalom's patient Ginny, for example, all is surface, with the fear that there is nothing underneath. She senses that she is going through the motions, that her life is an impersonation of life, that she's "flirting with a woman's identity" (Yalom and Elkin 1974, 24), writing at one point, "I have no spontaneous feelings. . . . Whenever I go outside, I feel fearful and must prepare myself" (xii). She depends on others, she writes, to "give me my setting and pulse." She states that she has felt at times in her life "both vibrant and dead" and that she "needed [others'] push. I could never be self-starting" (xx).

Singer describes his patients as even more cut off from object relations with others, relying not on others to give them a "setting and pulse," but on fragmentary feeling-states or sensations to "anchor" their identities. According to Singer, his patients use these feeling-states to create "false selves" to ward off the horror of feelings of inner emptiness or deadness. For some patients, any physical feeling, whether pleasant or unpleasant, can become a kind of anchor point to the external world, providing a partial sliver of existence in place of a sense of internal void.

Singer's and Yalom's patients, coming of age in the mid 1970s, bear a striking resemblance to some of the earliest documented cases thought to be borderline. Deutsch described the "as if" personality as showing a "completely passive attitude to the environment with a highly plastic readiness to pick up signals from the outer world and to mold oneself and one's behavior accordingly" (Deutsch, in Stone 1986, 77). Deutsch comments on the sense of superficiality that such patients showed, writing, "It is like the performance of an actor who is technically well trained but who lacks the necessary spark to make his impersonations true to life" (76).

One of Helene Deutsch's case illustrations of the "as if" personality is a patient she describes as "a pretty, temperamental woman of thirty-five with many intellectual and artistic talents," who comes to analysis "because she was 'tired' after a long series of adventures." Deutsch observes that such a motive masks a deep interest in psychoanalysis, and a wish to identify herself "with a 'particularly solid' professional personality"—that is, with Deutsch and her position as analyst. "Her plan was to become an analyst by identification with her analyst" (84). Deutsch states that while this patient has read widely on Freudian theory, "her understanding of them was extraordinarily superficial and her interest entirely unreal" (83). Such superficiality is "true not only for all her intellectual interests but for everything she did or had ever done. . . . All her experiences too were based on identifications . . . so many concurrent identifications—or symbolic representations of identifications—that her conduct appeared erratic. She was, in fact, considered 'crazy' by those who knew her" (84). When her plan of becoming an analyst proves impossible, the woman collapses. "She was completely lacking in affect and complained, 'I am so empty! My God, I am so empty! I have no feelings'" (84). Deutsch's patients, then, appear to be split between a superficial and a highly artificial performance that covers an underlying emptiness.

This theme of artificial surface performance is dramatically illustrated in the case of Ms. V., written by Martin Stein in 1989. This case illustrates the oscillations between masquerade and abjection that so frequently appear in the case narratives of borderline patients. Stein uses the metaphor of the mask to interpret the patient's behavior in therapy. He follows the contours of this performative masking behavior closely, and his rich description provides a glimpse of the terrain on which the connections between masking and gender relations and images can be charted.

The opening sentence provides several codes that locate and mark Ms. V. socially: She is a "35 year old Italian female who lives in a rent stabilized apartment in Brooklyn" (Stein 1989, 124). Ms. V. has recently left another therapist and sought a more experienced one. Stein then moves into the more detailed visual portrait of Ms. V.'s exaggerated feminine appearance. Her dress, excessive makeup, and clothing "gave her the appearance of a street walker, one ten to fifteen years younger than her stated age" (124). Here, her femininity implies for Stein not only a crude, lower-class appearance, but also a kind of artificial and monstrous or deathly image, captured in his depiction of her as the "vampire wife."

This theme is echoed by his comment that she appears to be the "dark daughter" in comparison to her sister, who is described as the "light daughter," with her contrast to Ms. V. depicted in a way that equates color with character, hence showing the racial codings of Stein's description. The sister is described as "very fair in complexion, blond, and married to a passive, malleable man" (126). As the "dark daughter," Ms. V. "represents the more primitive, antisocial, aggressive and perverse parts of the mother, while the sister is the externalization of the mother's more libidinally invested self representation" (126). Here Stein's narrative codes a hierarchy of values wherein darkness represents the primitive and savage, aggressive impulses, while light symbolizes goodness and passivity. Further, outward, visual appearance operates as a language that Stein uses to decide the mysteries of the patient's past. He compares Ms. V. to her mother, surmising that Ms. V. may be seen as a "distorted version of her," noting that "my seeing a picture of the patient's mother gave credence to this view" (126).

Patients deemed borderline are frequently those who transgress the boundaries of proper or appropriate social behavior, both inside and outside the therapy. In Ms. V.'s symptom list, social deviance figures prominently, including "excessive drinking and self destructive promiscuity," kleptomania, and poor or nonexistent personal hygiene. In addition to social deviance, the patient suffers from "problems with identity" with "contradictory self images, multiple unintegrated self representations and an inability to judge how she looks" (125). Stein, as Singer and Chessick do with their patients, traces Ms. V.'s instability to her early relationship to her mother, but also includes her relationship to her father as a secondary theme in his interpretation of her "developmental deficits."

In the discussion of what Stein calls a "therapeutic odyssey," Stein describes the difficult, tumultuous course of therapy. Like other patients diagnosed as borderline, Ms. V. tests the boundaries of the therapeutic relationship, phoning him at all hours, and "calculated how long it took me to respond" (130). At one point she asks Stein to write a letter to the public library absolving her of her library fines, and becomes enraged when he refuses. Stein writes that she is dependent on Stein, and yet tries to "control and manipulate" him. She expresses doubts about his love and concern for her, and "lamented that this was just a job for me. How could she really ever trust me and be sure of my 'sincerity'?" (130). Stein notes that he avoids countertransference anger or frustration by using humor to defuse the intensity of her demands.

Stein traces such demands to her relationship with her mother, and ultimately to the early development and structure of her self. Her mother has simultaneously "rescued" her and devalued her, and it is out of this early relationship that the patient forms a negative self-image. Her attempts to control her therapist mimic her mother's treatment of her. "All these variables spoke to serious developmental deficits in this patient" (129). Stein encourages a separation from the mother, and the narrative traces the progress of that separation.

The theme of promiscuity and abusive relationships with men is central to the narrative as it unfolds. Indeed, the most important symptom listed by Stein involves "transient relationships with abusive men often leading to physical abuse and precarious situations," which Stein refers to as "self-destructive." Further, Stein writes, "The patient appeared to induce or invite such sadistic behavior in these men" (125). Stein notes that she has an "obsession with finding a man to marry her and ruminating about this" (125). Yet she also protests against the way men devalue her. Stein writes that in "one session the patient complained 'why do all these men use me? . . . Why don't they like me for me?'"

Stein's response could be perceived as a form of victim blaming and echoes the problem of faulting victims of abuse or sexual assault for their "provocative dress": "I responded by stating 'Maybe it's because of the way you look!'" (127) Perhaps her dress, he goes on, gives men the message that sex is all that she is looking for. This comment effectively translates her own verbal protest about her position in gender relations, in which she is devalued and demeaned, into a symptom of a psychological disturbance, and ultimately to an unstable self or ego that must be shored up. He states that he feels he is functioning as an "auxiliary ego" in "demonstrating the relation between appearance, behavior, and the consequences of such" (128).

Stein's focus on Ms. V.'s "provoking" men's violence is troubling and indeed may obscure the sources of her psychic disturbance. Stein dwells on these aspects of her situation near the beginning of the case narrative. However, as the story unfolds his attention shifts away from her provocative behavior and toward another story: the drama of Ms. V.'s split self, and Stein's discovery of her creation of symbolic "masks" to cover her inner sense of emptiness.

During the second year of treatment, an interesting ritual emerges during the sessions: The patient begins taking out a makeup mirror and putting on skin and eye makeup while speaking to Stein. Ms. V. begins to speak about the significance of putting on makeup as a form of creating a "face," and speaks of the different "faces" that she creates through her makeup. Ms. V. says that when she is alone, to stave off feelings of emptiness and anxiety she stands in front of a mirror and applies makeup. She tells Stein that she never washes her makeup off, simply applying another layer onto the existing one. "This amounted to her putting on a 'mask' in the morning, on top of the previous day's. The thought of being without make-up terrified her" (132).

Enacting the makeup ritual in therapy leads her to make associations between her surface, facial appearance and "deeper feelings and experience: that is from surface to depth" (131). Ms. V. tells Stein that she is never sure what she looks like under her makeup. She feels that the more makeup she wears, the better she looks. Stein interprets this to be saying that she doesn't know "who she [is]" and that the makeup is a way of creating a self (132). "One thing was certain through her facial make-up, she created a sense of self and identity, mirroring a process that should go on internally. Furthermore, it was an identity so fragile that it could be washed away in the morning" (134).

While viewing her behavior in therapy as inappropriate, Stein allows it to continue since he feels it is a significant reflection of her inner lack of cohesive self. Putting on makeup helps her avoid "possible loss of identity, depersonalization, or even transient psychosis" (131). Stein uses the metaphor of the mask to represent her creation of faces. The creation of an outer mask, says Stein, serves as an outward "binding" of her self in the face of its possible dissolution.

> In many primitive and ancient cultures, the actors wore masks while performing, so that the true self and emotions of the characters they were playing could emerge. . . . I had the strong conviction that this patient was communicating very compli-cated and frightening affects via symbolic representation. Likewise, as alluded to earlier, the "faces" that she created seemed to have a "binding" function, a transitional identity, if you will, which the patient created to avoid possible fragmenta-tion and depersonalization as deeper parts of her personality were explored. (132)

Later in the therapy the patient reveals to Stein that she rarely washes, and never washes her clothes, wearing all of them, including undergarments, until they have to be thrown away. At one point she confides in Stein, "When I find a man who loves me I'll wash!" (133) Stein elaborates on his reactions to her revelations: "I had many pri-vate associations to the patient's verbalizations. Wearing her make-up at night brought up images of a corpse, symbolic of her inner empti-ness and emotional 'deadness,' (she was not orgasmic during inter-course). I thought of a skunk's self protective odor and her not washing as a possible distancing mechanism. . . . I also thought of her not wash-ing a variation of a 'hunger strike' or a state similar to anorexia "I won't eat until someone loves me!" (133).

Ms. V. makes a direct connection to gender relations and to her makeup and dress as a way of performing a heterosexualized feminin-ity, stating that she wears excessive makeup and "provocative" cloth-ing to get men to notice her. Without this outward mask or performance, she feels she is "invisible/worthless" to others.

As Singer does with his patients, Stein fits Ms. V.'s behavior into the developmental story lines of the normal self in early infancy. Stein's interpretation connects her current rituals to her early relationship with her mother (and later, father). He suggests that Ms. V.'s mother envied her and devalued her, and that the patient has internalized these hostile feelings as a part of the self, her "maternal introject" in which a fantasized image of the mother is incorporated into the psyche: "Was her not washing a reflection of rage at her maternal introject in a manner similar to 'starving' a hated introject, or a symbolic expression of how she felt about herself on a deep level?" (133).

As Stein and Ms. V. discuss these interpretations, Stein notices that her dress and makeup become "toned down" and less flamboyant, while at the same time, she begins to assert herself toward her mother. Stein notes, "I felt that this was to a large degree due to more internal structuralization" (135). Another pattern is her growing self-valuation, as she begins to focus on protecting and supporting herself in relationships. The narrative describes Ms. V.'s growing confidence and healthy self-regard, and the apparent success of the therapy.

In spite of this apparent success, as the second year of her therapy draws to a close, the patient abruptly terminates her therapy, stating in a phone message that she wants to find a woman therapist. Stein's bewildered reaction is reflected in his writing in the case account, "What happened!" He considers several explanations, including the possibility that perhaps she is ready to end therapy and that he should have raised the issue. He also considers her ambivalent feelings about her father, which had emerged with particular intensity at their last session. She felt wounded at her father's abandonment of her, and felt a sense of loss of his love.

Yet it is Stein's closing question that brings the gender politics of the case to the forefront. Speculating on the mystery of why Ms. V. has terminated her treatment, Stein writes, "In closing, there is one more troubling fact, that can only be speculated about. Was Ms. V. sexually abused? . . . She had very few memories of her childhood, and perhaps her sudden exit from therapy was due to the possible emergence of such memories and the anxiety/rage associated with such a trauma" (138). The question, coming as it does at the end of his account, and without being developed as a theme in the narrative, appears to be an afterthought, directed more to the question of her termination of therapy rather than to her psychic troubles. Posed too late in the case and in the narrative, it appears to have the potential to offer a different trajectory to the analysis. Yet Stein is left with only an unfinished analysis and many questions. Stein's question may also reflect a reaction to

Ms. V.'s wanting a woman therapist, though he doesn't explicitly address this.

Lost Self: Ginny

We can gain further insight into the theme of fragmented subjectivity from examining two cases that focus heavily on this theme. These include the case of Ginny, as depicted both by the patient herself and by her psychotherapist, Irving Yalom, in a cowritten case account published in 1974, as well as the case of Laurie, a case analyzed by Jane Flax from a feminist perspective.

Like Singer and Stein, Yalom and Flax describe their borderline patients as having split selves. Yet the interpretation these therapists offer of the origin and workings of this split is very different. Each of them situates these splits, not in the pre-oedipal relationship to the mother, but in the social milieu within which feminine selfhood is constructed. These authors show in their narratives a recognition of the effects of gender borders and the power of dominant images of femininity on women's subjectivity and construction of self.

A case history of the psychotherapy of a borderline patient is presented in *Every Day Gets a Little Closer: A Twice-Told Therapy*, coauthored by psychotherapist Irvin Yalom and his patient "Ginny Elkin" (Yalom and Elkin 1974). This case is explicitly jointly produced, with both Yalom and Elkin writing a series of postsession reports. The book is an outgrowth of the arrangement between Yalom and Elkin, who writes the accounts of their sessions as payment for therapy.

Elkin's borderline status is defined for the reader immediately, in the foreword by Yalom, who believes that "because of her ego boundary blurring, her autism, her dream life, the inaccessibility of affect, most clinicians would affix to her a label of 'schizoid' or, perhaps, 'borderline'" (xiv). This is corroborated later with the assessment of another therapist, who states that Elkin was "beleaguered by frightening masochistic sexual fantasies and manifestly borderline schizophrenic thought processes" (xv). She is described by the therapists who run the group therapy sessions she participates in: "ethereal . . . wistful . . . a haughty but self-conscious amusement at the whole proceedings . . . reality would never fully engage her energies . . . alternated between being someone who was extraordinarily sensitive and reactive to others, to someone who simply was not there at all . . . a mystery in the group . . . a borderline schizophrenic yet she never came close to the border of psychosis" (xvi).

This statement shows the mutable and shifting meaning of the borderline label, with its simultaneously close associations to, and distinction from, psychosis. It also signifies a marginal presence that refuses to be integrated within the group. Her distance from reality, her conscious invisibility ("not there at all"), indicate that she is simply inaccessible. She cannot be brought into the circle. She is placed linguistically at the border of madness, though "she never came close to the border of psychosis." Here we see the function of the borderline label, in enabling an inaccessible person to be understood as pathological, as outside the bounds of normality, without being declared psychotic.

After their first meeting, Elkin recounts her main difficulties in living "in a confusing and unsystematic fashion," and underneath her explicit complaints there is evidence of a "litany of self-hatred":

> She is masochistic in all things. All her life she has neglected
> her own needs and pleasures. She has no respect for herself. She
> feels she is a disembodied spirit—a chirping canary hopping
> back and forth from shoulder to shoulder, as she and her friends
> walk down the street. She imagines that only as an ethereal
> wisp is she of interest to others. . . . She is consumed with self-
> contempt. A small voice inside endlessly taunts her. Should she
> forget herself for a moment and engage life spontaneously, the
> pleasure-stripping voice brings her back sharply to her casket of
> self-consciousness. (xii)

Yalom recounts other symptoms: "She has no sense of herself"; she is unable to express anger (in contrast to many of the other cases of borderline disorder); she has "no rights" in Yalom's words; she is "consumed with self-contempt"; she has never been able to sustain a lasting relationship with a man; she has difficulty swallowing and in her teens vomited frequently; she has nightmares of sexual violation by women and men. "By the end of the hour I felt considerable alarm about Ginny. Despite many strengths—a soft charm, deep sensitivity, wit, a highly developed comic sense, a remarkable gift for verbal imagery—I found pathology wherever I turned: too much primitive material, dreams which obscured the reality-fantasy border, but above all a strange diffuseness, a blurring of 'ego boundaries'" (xiv).

How does Elkin present herself in her narrative? The tone of Elkin's narrative is one of irony and bemusement at herself. Unlike the depictions of Singer's patients, who describe an excruciating sense of emptiness, Elkin expresses a milder sense of dislocation and inability to fix herself. Her self descriptions suggest a detachment from both her surroundings and her self. She is unable to get a fix on her desires, and seems to be passively watching life pass. At one point she says, "I just shop a lot of attitudes and feelings without buying any" (143). Elkin appears to be searching for meaning and authenticity:

> I was an A student in high school in New York. Even though I was creative, that was just a sideline to being mostly stunned, as though I had been hit on the head by a monster shyness. I went through puberty with my eyes shut and my head migrained. Fairly early in my college life I put myself out to pasture academically. Although I did occasional "great" work, I like nothing better than to be a human sundial, a curled up outdoor nap. I was scared of boys and didn't have any. My few later affairs were all surprises. As part of my college education, I spent some time in Europe working and studying and compiling a dramatic résumé that was really all anecdotes and friends, not progress. What passed for bravery was a form of nervous energy and inertia. I was scared to go home. After I graduated from college, I returned to New York. I couldn't find a job, in fact had no direction. My qualifications dripped like Dali's watch, as I was tempted toward everything and nothing. (xix)

Two main themes are prominent in Elkin's accounts of the therapy; one is her sense of artificiality and detachment from others and from her emotions, and a second theme is her reaction to the rituals of therapy itself. Elkin defines herself as responding to others' initiatives rather than to her own: "I react to someone rather than act first. They put me in a place, set my borders and limits" (91). She describes an inability to feel strong emotions: "I know my problem has something to do with suspension of action and feeling" (82). This state of "suspension" is expressed in another entry, in which she writes, "What follows close behind me is my catatonic shadow that convinces me. . . . I do not move. . . . I do not stagger on. . . . I don't progress. . . . I only pose, a model for my shadow, a shadow for my silhouette" (50).

She survives through fantasy; as she writes after one therapy session, "This is how I deal with things. Fantasy is resilient. I had no expectations about the session. I went into it blind. I was fantasying so much I didn't even think about the session" (92). Elkin is particularly detached from anger, which Yalom encourages her to explore in her relationship to her boyfriend and to Yalom himself in therapy.

This detachment is apparent in her sense that therapy is contrived, artificial, and that she is performing, both in the session with Yalom, and in the write-ups:

> I say things in therapy that are not true. Even as I'm saying
> them, I know I don't believe them, that they will confuse you.
> Like when I said, "you're sitting across from me and seeing
> nothing." Many times you've told me you don't think of me as
> nothing. If only I could catch myself when I'm saying things
> like that, contradict myself, say "No that's not what I mean,"
> maybe then I could take myself seriously when I speak. I don't
> fight for my words. They just come. (54)

The problem seems to be language itself: "I really think I must be still burrowed in the cave, like Plato's cave, since I write and think only with analogies. Everything is like something else. Even this write-up is so veiled, it is not direct" (44).

Thus, Elkin appears to have no center; she is unfocused. While she appears more "tangible" than some of Singer's patients, she too lacks the firm stable self, the center of initiative and action, passively responding to the needs of others.

Yalom is concerned with her lack of self-assertion, particularly with her relationship to her boyfriend Karl. He writes of frustration when she tells him she is waiting for Karl to tell her when he will move out. Elkin, by contrast, prioritizes the relationship over her rights, stating, "I would do anything just to keep myself in a relationship. Even though I might be totally camouflaged, so the other person doesn't know I'm there" (28).

Yalom, like Singer, writes of his borderline patient's false outer self, which covers a suppressed inner state. Yalom, however, does not perceive this inner state as a void, but rather as an underlying autonomous self that is forbidden expression by other aspects of Elkin's self.

Yalom states that Elkin's main problem is self-effacement in her relationships to others, in order that she may gain, he writes, "love, and at any cost" (219). Elkin, writes Yalom, can never be loved enough. "She could never stop pressing herself to be better, more selfless, more pleasing" (220). To gain love and approval from others, Elkin, writes Yalom, "nurtured the hostess parts of herself, her amusing chirping wit, her generosity, her selflessness" (219). Her true self is suppressed—"rage, greed, self—assertiveness, independence and personal desire were all regarded as saboteurs to the regime of love—all were exiled to the remotest regions of her mind. They emerged only in impulsive, out-of-the-blue flashes or, heavily disguised, in fantasies and dreams" (220).

In addition to the suppressed "will" there is another self, Elkin's "inner critic," who legislates among her selves and actively suppresses her "will." Yalom says that this critical self is an "inner demon," a "pleasure stripping voice" inside her (220).

Thus, Yalom is sensitive to the complexities of Elkin's subjectivity and to some of the interpersonal forces that contribute to her feeling of emptiness and depersonalization. Yet he adheres to the intrapsychic focus of a developmental psychology and stresses that these dynamics of her interpersonal world are "irrational." He wants to tell her, he writes, "Your frantic search for love is irrational; it is a frozen piece of ancient behavior transported into the present, and ill-suited for your adult life. Your panic at the threat of love-withdrawal, appropriate no doubt in earliest infancy, is similarly irrational; you are capable of survival without stifling nurturance" (220).

Yet if Elkin's "problem" is not so much an internal negation of her will, but a subjective position in relation to cultural negation, in his exhortations Yalom underestimates the power of cultural forces that shape the construction of identity. At one point, in describing some of the behavioral techniques that he uses with Elkin, Yalom states, "She had an irrational fear (a phobia, if you will) of self-assertion. She acted as if some calamity would ensue were she to demand her rights or express anger or merely a conflicting opinion" (224). This statement, when considered in the context of real "calamity" faced by women who do demand their rights (at home, or in the public sphere of work or politics) minimizes cultural prohibitions and fails to consider Elkin's fears as an intelligible response to these prohibitions.

Yalom sets himself the task of opposing, he writes, "those forces that smothered her will" without linking those internal prohibitions to an acknowledgment of the societal prohibitions against women's anger and against which they construct selves. He is thus in the role of surrogate parent, an individual representative of society, with whom Elkin can relearn the boundaries and potentialities of her self.

The following case takes Yalom's analysis one step further, situating the subjective conflicts of the borderline patient in the context of gender relations.

Repressed Selves: The Case of Laurie

Jane Flax, in her discussion of Laurie, also notices the fragmentation of self and the phenomenon of a "false self" in her patient. Yet what is different about Flax's rendering of the split or fragmented self is that she situates this split self in a context of sociocultural gender relations. She analyzes her patient's fragmented identity as a discursive and cultural construction, thus making the connections between individual female experience and gender discourse.

In her discussion of her patient, Flax argues that Laurie's "core self" is split between an outward false self that conforms to the feminine role, and a repressed, split-off, autonomous self that is forbidden expression in contemporary Western culture. Thus, the source of the borderline patient's fragmented self is ultimately a cultural source: the construction of femininity in Western culture. The patient's borderline symptoms are expressions of the confusions, ambiguities, and contradictions faced by women as each of these parts of the self struggles for expression.

Jane Flax describes this duality of self in women:

> My clinical experience and reading convince me that the repressed *is* gendered in the sense that women in our culture tend to repress distinctive aspects of the self which are bound up with autonomy and aggression. One dimension of what is repressed is women's non-object related ambition and interest in exerting various sorts of mastery: interpersonal, intellectual,

or creative. Both men's and women's sense of gender and the
self partially grow out of and are dependent upon the repression
of women's desire and ambition. Both genders maintain an
active interest in forestalling or prohibiting the return of this
repressed material. (Flax 1986, 92)

The construction of the self as feminine creates a double bind, given
that if women are to be considered normal, they must suppress their
nonfeminine aspects: autonomy and aggression. Yet in order to enter
the realm of the subject, they must disavow their feminine embodiment:
"In order to be valuable persons worthy of esteem, women must control the body and access to it. The world of thought and action is the
world of men; to enter it women must leave their distinctively female
bodies and sexuality 'outside.' One cannot be both a sexual, embodied
woman and an esteemed thinker and effective actor in the world" (101).

This repression of the realm of the embodied feminine subject is
manifest, according to Flax, in her patient Laurie's split into a "mostly
false (but predominant) 'social self,'—the conforming, nurturant feminine self "that women are usually praised for" (98); and two repressed
selves, forbidden for women in Western culture: "an autonomous (and
highly underdeveloped) self, and a 'sexual' self (also underdeveloped,
but not as forbidden or constricted as the autonomous self)" (98). Such
splitting off of forbidden selves creates Laurie's borderline fragmentation: "In order to survive she split off parts of her self, protecting some
with rigid defenses and repressing others." Such denial and repression
create turmoil in Laurie's relationships with people and in her "internal worlds," which are marked by "rigidity, rage, terror, loneliness, self-
hate, and a (disavowed but desperate) need for love."

Flax notes that these conflicts are evident in Laurie's relationship
to her in the therapy: "Laurie fears that I will not give her what she
needs in order to grow and develop as a separate person (or that I will
actively inhibit her from doing so). Alternatively, she fears that I will
hate her for becoming her 'real self,' as Laurie believes every member
of her family did, each for their own distinct reasons" (97). This is an
example of the double bind of the engulfment/abandonment dilemma,
in which women who seek relationship with others face the risk of becoming engulfed in the other and of disappearing as separate selves, yet
fear being abandoned when they try to assert autonomy.

These realizations and fears emerge only after three years of therapy with Flax, however. Laurie is actively suicidal when she first begins seeing Flax, as a result of "having had such a fragmented and unintegrated self most of her life" (97). Early in her treatment with Flax, Laurie becomes actively suicidal and panic-stricken, even purchasing a gun. In response, Flax assists Laurie in seeking short-term hospitalization.

In the course of the subsequent therapy, Laurie's family background emerges, which Flax sees as a specific local instance of wider cultural prohibitions and contradictions for women's identity. Flax's reading of the causes of the borderline patient's psychic fragmentation and turbulence is oriented toward the cultural context within which women construct selves. "While the contents of Laurie's repressed [sic] can be understood by mapping out and locating them within her family dynamics, I think that her repressed material is widely shared by other women in Western culture. This commonality makes her case relevant to the more general questions of gender, repression, and subjectivity" (98).

Laurie, according to Flax, is enmeshed in a family and cultural milieu that demands her conformity with its demands; hence her false, nurturing and caretaking "social self" predominated at the cost of "the mutilation or denial of the other selves" (99). Flax argues, "The social self is the part of the self that women are usually praised for—it strives to satisfy the needs of others; it is capable of empathy; it desperately wants and needs interpersonal interaction" (98). Flax argues that Laurie plays this role as "echoes" of her family's own selves: "Here it is not the self which is to blame but the context in and conditions under which it comes to be and must exist (and how these conditions are taken into and become part of this self). In Laurie's case, her family wanted this part of her to exist only to service other people's needs, not her own. She could only be in relationships with her mother, father, or brother on their terms and as a means to their ends—symbiotic fusion for the mother, narcissistic echo for the father, scapegoat and actor-out of forbidden feelings for the brother" (99).

One of the "repressed" selves is the "sexual self." Flax traces the repression of this self directly to cultural perception of women's bodies, particularly in relation to hunger and sexuality, transmitted to Laurie by her parents. Laurie's mother "regarded the body as an enemy that needed to be regulated and controlled. . . . The dangers of the body were condensed, focused, and expressed through the mother's intense, persistent preoccupation with food and weight" (100). Her mother's control of Laurie's appearance and food consumption produced Laurie's anorexia and bulimia.

Laurie's father gave her similar messages about women's bodies as passive objects to be regulated. Her father's messages about sexuality portrayed women as passive objects or victims.

Flax provides a feminist reading of the effects of Laurie's internalization of such messages, in creating a fragmented identity split between body and mind, in which women are encouraged both to "become" a sexual object, and to deny this embodied sexuality in order to escape the fates of the body's appetites: "Thus Laurie learned that a woman's body is the site of danger, exploitation, and entrapment. Becoming a sexual being/object would be an impediment to or even irreconcilable with what really counts according to the father: the mind, abstract thought, and argument. . . . (Laurie has had persistent dreams of being punished, even hung by her father for becoming pregnant.) Even in sexuality, however, men are the active agents—women are the 'cause' of men's desire, but they have no independent or initiating desire of their own" (101).

Thus, Laurie's "domestic metaphysics" center on the assumption that "minds and bodies are two completely distinct entities" (103). Flax's interpretation makes a direct connection between Laurie's split borderline identity and the gendered, cultural split between the abstract mind and the uncontrolled body. Laurie appears caught in the double bind created by this duality: She cancels out her own desires in her regulation of her body's appearance, thereby meeting her family's and society's expectations to transform herself into a passive feminine (sexual) image or object, yet is warned of the dangers of this very acquisition of a feminine body. In order to enter her father's world, she must disembody herself. Yet the overall message is the cancellation of Laurie's autonomous desires. Thus, Laurie cancels out her autonomous selfhood because she wants to be accepted into the world and to meet her family's (and society's) expectations.

More forbidden than the sexual self is Laurie's repressed "autonomous self." "Laurie believes this to be the most 'mutilated' and underdeveloped of her three selves. She likens it to the binding of feet—the toes curled under and deformed—to render woman helpless and pleasing to men" (104). The autonomous self, in Flax's words, "would enjoy mastery, aggression, competition, and define its desires independently of, even against, the wishes of others" (105). And yet, Flax is concerned lest this self begin to resemble the sort of rigid, bounded self that feminist theory has identified as "masculinist": "By autonomous, however, Laurie (and I) do not mean a self that denies its embeddedness in many kinds of social relations. For a notion of autonomy that is opposed to the 'social' or to 'connection to others' is itself a barrier to the development and enjoyment of such a self" (104). For Flax, the "autonomous self" denied women is neither the fully relational nurturant self, congruent with cultural definitions of femininity, nor the "'unitary,' mentalist, deeroticized, masterful, and oppositional" self that is congruent with cultural definitions of masculinity (93). The autonomous self that Laurie's family and her culture won't allow her access to is defined by Flax as transcending such gendered splits between dependence or engulfment on one hand and isolation and separation on the other.

Clearly, Flax's feminist orientation enables her to "see," and to help Laurie discover, this feminist self. It is a utopian self, since, as Flax states, it does not and cannot yet exist in contemporary culture, due to the powerful forces of repression at work that mitigate against such selfhood for women. Flax moves from a discussion of Laurie to a general discussion of this ideal self and the collective feminist action that would enable its emergence. "By retrieving repressed aspects of the self together—our anger, our connections with, attractions to, and fear of other women, our self-hate—we also begin to find in this 'new' memory a powerful impulse toward political actions. Experiences in therapy and consciousness raising confirm that memory in its fullness requires access to the various aspects of the self" (106).

Thus, Flax locates Laurie's fragmentation within the wider cultural splits and fragmentations that influence women's construction of identity. As a feminist, Flax is oriented not only to early childhood experiences and relationships, but to cultural prohibitions and repressions and their psychic and bodily costs for women. Borderline subjectivity, then, is potentially the subjectivity of all Western women, crystallizing in particularly intense form in borderline patients such as Laurie through an especially extreme degree of repression by her family. Yet Flax's perspective is "pre-Foucaultian" in that it does not address the problem of new forms of power that work to produce forms of selfhood, rather than repress them. Her perspective would thus be unable to explain the ways women actively produce themselves as gendered beings, within the commodification of images of femininity.

Thus, as in Singer's and Chessick's analyses of borderline cases, the immediate site of contestation that has major consequences for the borderline patient's fragmentation of self is relationships—specifically, the family. Each member has reinforced and prejudiced this construction of split selfhood in relation to Laurie. The difference here, however, is that Flax explicitly addresses the wider context within which the family is situated, and the means by which the family transmits cultural messages to women.

Borderline Double: The Case of Marge

The case of Marge, described by Irving Yalom in "Therapeutic Monogamy" (1989), is a dramatic illustration of the performative masking of the feminine, but here in the form of an alternate personality, a dark, seductive double who emerges as a shadow side to the passive, reclusive borderline patient, Marge. We can also see, in Yalom's evocative narrative rendering of this dramatic fragmentation, a textual magnification of this fragmentation.

In introducing the reader to Marge, Yalom acknowledges his immediate dread of her when they first meet, as he recognizes that she may very well be a borderline: "It didn't take much experience to recognize the signs of deep distress. Her sagging head and shoulders said 'depression'; her gigantic eye pupils and restless hands and feet said 'anxiety.' Everything else about her—multiple suicide attempts, eating disorder, early sexual abuse by her father, episodic psychotic thinking, twenty-three years of therapy—shouted 'borderline,' the word that strikes terror in the heart of the middle-aged comfort-seeking psychiatrist" (Yalom 1989, 213).

At the next therapy session, Marge speaks "like a simulacrum—with uncanny stillness, with nothing moving but her lips, not her breath, or her hands, or her eyes, or even her cheeks." "I am forty-five years old. I have been mentally ill all my life. I have seen psychiatrists since I was twelve years old and cannot function without them. I shall have to take medicine the rest of my life. The most I can hope for is to stay out of a mental hospital. I have never been loved. I will never have children. . . . My father, who molested me when I was a child, is dead. My mother is a crazy, embittered lady, and I grow more like her every day" (216).

Yalom writes that the "simulacrum" speaking is not exactly the woman, Marge, but a tormented part of her: "It was her depression speaking." In an effort to give back Marge's "self" to her, Yalom reads back to her one of her own letters that she had sent to him, in effect giving her back her own self-narrative, which she has lost. Marge appears visibly improved. This seemingly "healthy self," however, dissolves three weeks later, when Marge undergoes a transformation: "In the middle of her dirge, she suddenly closed her eyes—not in itself unusual since she often went into an autohypnotic state during the session. . . . I said, 'Marge,' and was about to utter the rest of the sentence, 'Will you please come back?' when I heard a strange and powerful voice come out of her mouth: 'You don't know me.' . . . The voice was so different, so forceful, so authoritative, I looked around the office for an instant to see who else might have entered. 'Who are you?' I asked. 'Me! Me!'" (222).

The emergence of Marge's monstrous double creates a nausea in Yalom, as he evokes the experience of witnessing the "forbidden": "For a brief time I felt a wave of eerie nausea, as though I were peering through a rent in the fabric of reality, at something forbidden, at the raw ingredients, the clefts and seams, the embryonic cells and blastulas that are, in the natural order of things, not meant to be seen in the finished human creature" (222).

Yet in spite of his nausea, Yalom is also riveted by Marge's performance. The narrative evokes vividly Yalom's response to Marge's double, and this narrative evocation constructs Me, the second self, as a seductive, powerful, yet threatening woman, whom Yalom calls a "Lorelei". In this narrative, therefore, Yalom constructs the borderline's fragmented self in highly gendered terms, reproducing the cultural split between passive femininity and forbidden sexual autonomy. Yalom is attracted to Me, and in the narrative draws out his own associations to this powerful double. The image of the beautiful woman as both seductive and deadly is openly embraced in his narrative:

This new Marge was vivacious and outrageously, but enjoyably, flirtatious. She was savvy, willful, very sexy. What a relief to have a break from Marge's droning voice and relentless whining. But I was beginning to feel uneasy; I enjoyed this lady too much. I thought of the Lorelei legend, and though I knew it would be dangerous to tarry, still I visited awhile. . . . Perhaps I was staying longer with her than I should. It was wrong to talk to her about Marge. It was not fair to Marge. Yet this woman's appeal was strong, almost irresistible. (222)

Yalom is captivated by Marge's double, which creates a dilemma for him: Marge is split, with two selves; which of her selves is he treating? Which self is "real"? "I felt bewildered by what had happened. My one basic rule—'Treat Marge as an equal' was no longer sufficient. Which Marge? The whimpering Marge in front of me or the sexy, insouciant Marge?" (224).

Yalom struggles with the question not only of which self is real, but also of which self he has a relationship to; he is concerned about being faithful to his patient, about "fidelity": "Above all I must not permit myself to be seduced by that other Marge."

Yalom interprets Marge's double as a false creation of her father, caused by his sexual abuse. Yalom is therefore wary of falling into the role of father in relation to this seductive yet artificial feminine self: "My implicit contract with Marge (as with all my patients) is that when I am with her, I am wholly, wholeheartedly, and exclusively with her. Marge illuminated another dimension of that contract: that I must be with her most central self. Rather than relating to this integral self, her father, who abused her, had contributed to the development of a false, sexual self. I must not make that error" (225).

Thus, Yalom advocates "Marge" as the real, central self, the integral self, and "Me"—the seductive powerful Other—as false, a creation of an incestuous relation to her father, a literal creation of patriarchal fantasy. Yet Yalom is nonetheless seemingly under this powerful double's spell. Staying faithful to Marge is difficult: "It was not easy. To be truthful, I wanted to see 'Me' again. Though I had known her for less than an hour I had been charmed by her. The drab backdrop of the dozens of hours I had spent with Marge made this engaging phantom stand out with a dazzling clarity" (225).

Yalom is not successful in preventing himself from re-creating the role of Marge's father in the creation of Me, as he expands on his own associations to this attractive "engaging phantom": "I didn't know her name and she didn't have much freedom, but we each knew how to find the other. In the next hour she tried several times to come to me again. I could see Marge flicker her eyelids and then close them. Only another minute or two, and we would have been together again. I felt foolish and eager. Balmy bygone memories flooded my mind. I recalled waiting at a palm-edged Caribbean airport for a plane to land and for my lover to join me" (225).

Me embodies not only the false Lorelei image, but the rage of that persona aimed against the other, passive self, Marge. Me says to Yalom, "You could have her in therapy for thirty years, but I'd still win. I can tear down a year's work in a day. If necessary, I could have her step off a curb into a moving truck. . . . Marge is a creep. You know she's a creep. How can you stand to be with her?" (223).

Me proceeds to parody Marge, providing, in Yalom's words, "an astounding theatrical performance," imitating Marge, her timidity, her fear, and despair. "It was a virtuoso performance. But also an unspeakably cruel performance by 'Me.' . . . Her eyes blazed as she continued to defile Marge who, she said, was incurable, hopeless, and pathetic" (223).

Me is not only alluring but also an "equal," in collusion with Yalom. "This woman, this 'Me,' she understood me. . . . She knew I wanted a real woman. . . . 'Me's' theatrical performance, in which she regurgitated all those snippets of Marge's behavior, convinced me that both she and I (and only she and I) understood what I had gone through with Marge. She was the brilliant, beautiful director who had created this film. . . . If she could play all those roles, she must be the concealed, guiding intelligence behind them all. We shared something that was beyond language" (225).

As this example shows, "Me" is a narrative construction, created by Yalom's graphic and vivid rendering of the eruption of the "beautiful and intriguing, but also lethal"—Me. With his attraction to Me, Yalom projects the image of the powerful and dangerous seductress onto Marge's performance. As depicted in the text, he "sees" Lorelei when

Marge's other personality emerges. Yalom's countertransferential captivation and fascination with Me finds its way into the text. Thus, the split Yalom describes for us is partly Yalom's own creation.

The title of the piece, "Therapeutic Monogamy," encapsulates the metaphor of therapy as marriage and fidelity to Marge, and the emergence of Me as a seductive figure, an "other woman," who conjures up Yalom's romantic fantasies. Clearly, these figures are intentionally exaggerated by Yalom for effect. Yet this metaphor of fidelity and temptation appears to magnify the dual images of women that constructed the Marge/Me split; the shrinking pathetic Marge, versus the beautiful and lethal seductress, Me. Yalom tells the story of continuing faithful to Marge, and keeping Me at bay, in spite of his temptation, and in spite of Me's "gathering strength and desperately trying to return to me."

Yalom's therapeutic ritual is aimed at bringing together these mutually exclusive opposites, to "establish a confederacy or fusion of the two Marges. . . . I would sacrifice her rival to her, pluck her feathers, pull her asunder, and, bit by bit, feed her to Marge. The feeding technique was to repeat one standard question: 'Marge, what would "she" say if she were here?'" (226).

The expectation is that a reconciliation of these conflicting personalities can be expected to occur within the bounds of Marge's "integral self"—her "most central self." Yalom "feeds" Me—the empowered, yet forbidden self—to Marge, in hopes that Marge will "ingest" or "appropriate" the best aspects of Me, while neutralizing her destructive power.

Yet from a feminist perspective, Marge's split self can be understood as the embodiment or personification, in exaggerated form, of the dual image of women in Western perception, a duality that makes the passive, subordinate "shrinking" Marge irreconcilable with the powerful Me. The double, Me, appears to carry all of Marge's power, self-assertion, and sexuality. These aspects of Marge are split off and embodied in another persona. They are prevented from being part of Marge's personality, not solely as the result of Marge's mental pathology but as a prohibition in the culture against women's power. Thus, the split between Marge and Me is a creation of her culture, a contradiction in the construction of gender, literalized in Marge's relationship to her father.

Yalom wants the integration of this feminine duality—a cultural projection of the passive-powerful images of women, the double bind within which Marge constructs her self—to occur at the individual, rather than the cultural level. This expectation speaks less to the limits of Yalom's own intentions than it does to the limits of the goal of a therapeutic reconciliation of the cultural contradiction of current gender relations.

Narrating the Borders: Autobiographical Accounts

> In telling his or her story, a person names the experience, and so establishes the discourse from which any explanation proceeds. Explanation may be framed as a search for meaning, a problem in relatedness, or as a cry of outrage against abuse or oppression. . . . Insofar as the essence of madness is silence, narrative offers an antidote. (Susko 1994, 102, 105)

> Freud neglected to ask how a woman comes into possession of her own story, becomes a subject, when even narrative convention assigns her the place of an object of desire. How does an object tell a story? (Kahane 1985, 21)

There is another perspective on the emptiness, numbness, depersonalization, and split selfhood depicted in the case narratives that can be gained by exploring autobiographical accounts by women receiving this diagnosis. In this section I examine two autobiographical memoirs: Susanna Kaysen's *Girl, Interrupted* (Kaysen 1993) and Jane Wanklin's *Let Me Make It Good: A Chronicle of My Life with Borderline Personality Disorder* (Wanklin 1997). While both of these accounts were published in the 1990s, Kaysen's focuses on events that happened in 1968, when she was eighteen; while Wanklin's focuses primarily on the 1980s and early 1990s. Kaysen's account is focused on her single hospital stay when she was eighteen, and on feelings of depersonalization, numbness, and depression. Wanklin's autobiography, written after borderline personality disorder was redefined in the DSM in the direction of the "angry, self-damaging" behaviors (Stone, in Cauwels 1992, 243) describes experiences of abuse, self-mutilation, and suicide attempts. Wanklin, diagnosed as borderline in the early 1990s, describes more than a decade of repeated hospitalizations, suicide attempts, anorexia, substance abuse, convulsive episodes of rage in the hospital, and episodes of self-cutting. These accounts illustrate how the borderline diagnosis was applied differently in the 1960s than it was in the 1990s, as well as providing a glimpse into the thoughts and experiences of women diagnosed as borderline in two different eras.

If illness, in Stephen Marcus's words, is in part "suffering from an incoherent story or an inadequate narrative account of oneself," then Kaysen and Wanklin attempt to reconstruct that coherence through their stories. Michael Susko points out that when persons suffering mental distress tell their stories, "what might otherwise be seen as isolated and senseless symptoms of distress reveal themselves to be meaningful parts of a person's life story" (Susko 1994, 101). In their accounts of their lives, they strive to explain and account for their actions, particularly their self-mutilation or suicide attempts.

Their narratives also repeatedly return to the question of the borders between sanity and madness. Kaysen writes, "I wasn't convinced I was crazy, though I feared I was. Some people say that having any conscious opinion on the matter is a mark of sanity, but I'm not sure that's true. I still think about it. I'll always have to think about it" (Kaysen 1993, 159). Both women talk back to their diagnoses. Kaysen includes the definition of borderline personality disorder from the DSM-III in her book. "So these were the charges against me" she muses. "It's a fairly accurate picture of me at eighteen, minus a few quirks like reckless driving and eating binges. . . . I'm tempted to try refuting it, but then I would be open to the further charges of 'defensiveness' and 'resistance'" (150).

Jane Wanklin is less equivocal. When informed that she was not, as previously thought, schizophrenic but has borderline personality disorder, she is incredulous. "All of a sudden, I no longer had the 'prestige' of being safely insane and worthy of a certain amount of quirky 'respect.' I was now listed as being on some borderline of a ridiculous sham of a 'diagnosis' that made me sound insignificant and disgusting" (Wanklin 1997, 283). Wanklin is outraged at the loss of her status as "safely insane," recognizing the pejorative overtones of the diagnosis of borderline personality disorder.

Kaysen and Wanklin perceive the question of their madness and their borderline diagnosis very differently. While Kaysen questions the definitions of normality and mental disorder within which she is classified, Wanklin searches for the origins of her more volatile disturbance in her early childhood, eventually accepting her diagnosis when she discovers that it has such an origin.

Living in Suspended Animation: Girl, Interrupted

In 1968, when she was eighteen years old, Susanna Kaysen was hospitalized for what became a nearly two-year stay in McLean Psychiatric Hospital, with a diagnosis of borderline personality disorder. Her narrative deals directly with the politics of knowledge and power within which she became judged as mad, and with her coming to terms with her identity as "mental hospital patient." Calling her diagnosis and hospitalization "one moment made to stand still and to stand for all the other moments" (Kaysen 1993, 167), Kaysen even includes a chapter entitled "My Diagnosis" in which she examines the meaning of borderline personality disorder with reference to her own life.

Kaysen's memoir is thus not only an account of her stay in the hospital, but also a dialogue with the psychiatric frameworks of meaning that have defined her as borderline. She was able to obtain her case record from McLean and incorporates portions of it into the book. Indeed, the book opens with the first page of her case folder, as though inviting readers into the case record.

Included from the case record is the referral form from the staff person who admitted her. Under "Reason for referral," appears, "Needed McLean for 3 yrs, increasing patternless [sic] of life, promiscous [sic], might kill self or get pregnant" (11). The equivalence given to suicide and pregnancy, with both of them posed as equivalent destructive termini to a young woman's life, starkly illustrates how norms of proper femininity shape norms of psychic stability. Here, psychiatric hospitalization is a means of control of Kaysen's presumed "promiscuity."

Kaysen was referred to McLean after a brief interview with a psychiatrist. She writes of her admission, "Perhaps it's still unclear how I ended up in there. . . . I didn't mention that I'd never seen that doctor before, that he decided to put me away after only fifteen minutes. Twenty, maybe. What about me was so deranged that in less than half an hour a doctor would pack me off to the nuthouse?" (39)

Her admission was a voluntary one, and yet Kaysen points out that she was not aware that she had the right to refuse admission at the time: "I signed myself in. I had to, because I was of age. It was that or a court order, though they could never have gotten a court order against me. I didn't know that, so I signed myself in" (39).

Kaysen reflects at length on the kind of perceptions and experiences she had that seemed poised on the "shimmering, ever-shifting borderline that like all boundaries beckons and asks to be crossed" (159). Kaysen, as Susan Cheever writes, "lets the line between sanity and craziness become so blurred in 'Girl, Interrupted' that often the patients at McLean seem rational and the nurses and authorities crazy" (Cheever 1993, 20).

What emerges in Kaysen's descriptions of her perceptions is a theme of depersonalization, numbness and emptiness. Kaysen's memoir uses a set of spatial metaphors to depict this blurred border between sanity and madness, naming the realm of madness the "parallel universe": "There are so many of them: worlds of the insane, the criminal, the crippled, the dying, perhaps of the dead as well. These worlds exist alongside this world and resemble it, but are not in it" (Kaysen 1993, 5). She slips through one of the "perforations in the membrane between here and there" (5), where she looks at the world from a strange new vantage point.

Kaysen describes her shift in perspective from the vantage point of the parallel universe. She begins seeing patterns in ordinary objects, "potential representations" within things, or alternatively she becomes unable to maintain the perceptual pattern of faces. Yet she makes clear that these are not hallucinations, but simply new ways of looking at the world. "It was my misfortune—or salvation—to be at all times perfectly conscious of my misperceptions of reality. I never 'believed' anything I saw or thought I saw" (41).

Kaysen also has an altered perception of her self and her own body. She describes a profound alienation from her body and fights against a sense that she does not exist as a flesh-and-blood person. During one episode she stares at her hand, concerned first that it appears "simian," and then fearing that there are no bones underneath the skin. She bites and scratches her hand to "try to get to the bottom of this" (103). "I wanted to see that my hand was a normal human hand, with bones" (102). Her search is cut short when other patients call in the staff nurse.

When she declares to the nurse that she is "not safe," she is given a heavy dose of Thorazine.

From Kaysen's point of view, her emptiness is a response to her lack of fit into the narrow roles society offered white middle-class privileged girls. Mixed with her resistance to these roles is a sense of inadequacy. "As far as I could see, life demanded skills I didn't have. The result was chronic emptiness and boredom. . . . Emptiness and boredom: what an understatement. What I felt was complete desolation. Desolation, despair, and depression" (156–157).

Kaysen writes that her madness is a form of resistance: "My ambition was to negate. The world, whether dense or hollow, provokes only my negations. When I was supposed to be awake, I was asleep; when I was supposed to speak, I was silent; when a pleasure offered itself to me, I avoided it. My hunger, my thirst, my loneliness and boredom and fear were all weapons aimed at my enemy, the world. . . . All my integrity seemed to lie in saying 'No'" (42).

Kaysen acknowledges that in part, she was willing to be incarcerated as a part of this refusal. "It was a very big No—the biggest No this side of suicide" (42).

In an account written two decades later for Janice Cauwels's *Imbroglio* (1992), Esther, a twenty-three-year-old patient in a special unit for borderline patients, describes feelings of alienation and estrangement from society's routines and bureaucratic obligations. Esther's account echoes Kaysen's "negation" and refusal to fit into the roles society offered her: "I don't want to be so many things. I don't want to be a brain surgeon, or a cafeteria worker. All my jobs I didn't want to do. . . . I feel really awful when I see my friends who know what they want. I'm nothing" (112). Her refusal seems a partial solution to her confusion: "Basically I've decided that I'm never doing anything so that nobody ever expects anything ever. No, really. I told my therapist I can't stand another failure" (113).

The lack of place and position for Kaysen and her feelings of desolation led to a suicide attempt prior to her hospitalization. She swallowed fifty aspirin and passed out in a supermarket in front of the meat counter. Significantly, she explains her act as a war between aspects of herself. She describes her subjectivity as being, like the meat at the meat counter, "bruised, bleeding, and imprisoned in a tight wrapping" (38). "I wanted to get rid of a certain aspect of my character. I was performing a kind of self-abortion with those aspirin" (39). After having her stomach pumped, she feels she has succeeded, if only temporarily: "I felt good. I wasn't dead, yet something was dead" (38).

Kaysen also describes a symptom that is extremely common for contemporary cases of borderline disorder: self-mutilation. "I spent hours in my butterfly chair banging my wrist. I did it in the evenings, like homework. . . . I banged the inside, where the veins converge. It swelled and turned a bit blue, but considering how hard and how much I banged it, the visible damage was slight" (153). She interprets her wrist-banging as a way to make tangible an abstract psychological pain. In her explanation Kaysen expands upon the DSM description of self-mutilation: "This behavior may . . . counteract feelings of 'numbness' and depersonalization that arise during periods of extreme stress. . . . I was trying to explain my situation to myself. My situation was that I was in pain and nobody knew it; even I had trouble knowing it. So I told myself, over and over, You are in pain. It was the only way I could get through to myself ('counteract feelings of "numbness"'). I was demonstrating, externally and irrefutably, an inward condition" (153).

While she is in the hospital, she comes to the realization that she wants to be a writer. She tells a social worker, "A writer . . . I'm going to be a writer" (133). Her social worker's response is to suggest that she become a dental technician. "I didn't like her because she didn't understand that this was me, and I was going to be a writer; I was not going to type term bills or sell au gratin bowls or do any other stupid things. She didn't like me because I was arrogant and uncooperative and probably still crazy for insisting on being a writer" (133).

The question of her future is answered with a marriage proposal. Ironically, it is both the ticket out of the hospital (Kaysen wryly comments, "In 1968, everybody could understand a marriage proposal" [133]) and the end of her sense of having a future or identity as a writer. When one of the other hospital patients asks, "What's going to happen then, after you're married?" she says, "Nothing. It's quiet. It's like— I don't know. It's like falling off a cliff. . . . I guess my life will just stop when I get married" (136).

Yet later in her life, she discovers a place for herself as a writer. "Boyfriends and literature: How can you make a life out of those two things? As it turns out, I did. . . . Back then I didn't know that I—or anyone— could make a life out of boyfriends and literature" (155).

Kaysen includes the DSM-III definition of borderline personality disorder, followed by the chapter "My Diagnosis." "What does borderline personality mean, anyhow?" she writes. "It appears to be a way station between neurosis and psychosis: a fractured but not disassembled psyche." She receives a decidedly different definition from a psychiatrist she sees after hospitalization: 'It's what they call people whose lifestyles bother them'" (151). Kaysen acknowledges the uncertain status of the borderline diagnosis as less than that of a mental illness: "If my diagnosis had been bipolar illness, for instance, the reaction to me and to this story would be slightly different. That's a chemical problem, you'd say to yourself, manic-depression, Lithium, all that. I would be blameless, somehow. And what about schizophrenia—that would send a chill up your spine. After all, that's real insanity. People don't 'recover' from schizophrenia. You'd have to wonder how much of what I'm telling you is true and how much imagined" (151).

Kaysen's reaction to the symptom of "instability of self-image, interpersonal relationships, and mood . . . uncertainty about . . . long-term goals or career choice" is to view such conflicts as endemic to adolescent experience: "Isn't this a good description of adolescence? Moody, fickle, faddish, insecure: in short, impossible" (152). She challenges the normative, yet arbitrary judgments of her personality as "unstable": "My self-image was not unstable. I saw myself, quite correctly, as unfit for the educational and social systems. But my parents and teachers did not share my self-image. Their image of me was unstable, since it was out of kilter with reality and based on their needs and wishes" (155).

When addressing the predominance of women among those diagnosed as borderline, she writes, "Note the construction of that sentence. They did not write, 'The disorder is more common in women.' It would still be suspect, but they didn't even bother trying to cover their tracks. Many disorders, judging by the hospital population, were more commonly diagnosed in women. Take, for example, 'compulsive promiscuity.' How many girls do you think a seventeen-year-old boy would have to screw to earn the label 'compulsively promiscuous?'" (157).

Noting that her discharge sheet from the hospital reads "Recovered," she writes, "Recovered. Had my personality crossed over that border, whatever and wherever it was, to resume life within the confines of the normal? Had I stopped arguing with my personality and learned to straddle the line between sane and insane?" (154).

The narrative ends with her encounter with the Vermeer painting *Girl, Interrupted at Her Music*, and her identification with the image of the girl in the painting: "Interrupted at her music: as my life had been, interrupted in the music of being seventeen, as her life had been, snatched and fixed on canvas: one moment made to stand still and to stand for all the other moments, whatever they would be or might have been. What life can recover from that?" (167).

Kaysen's identification with the image—as representation of a life "snatched and fixed"—invokes the meaning of madness as lifelong stigma, the power of madness as signifier to color and shape her life, to represent and constitute her identity. Gazing at the girl in the painting, Kaysen imagines that the girl is looking for recognition. "She was looking out, looking for someone who would see her" (167). Kaysen recalls the first time she had seen the painting, when she was seventeen. Her English teacher had taken her to the Frick Museum, and was later to initiate an affair with her. She imagines that the girl in the painting is issuing a warning: "Her mouth was slightly open, as if she had just drawn a breath in order to say to me, 'Don't!' . . . 'Wait,' she was saying, 'wait! Don't go!'" (166). This time, she tells her current lover, "'Don't you see, she's trying to get out.'" Kaysen writes, "I had something to tell her now. 'I see you.' I said" (167).

Kaysen's account shows her living at odds with normative femininity, in her sexual behavior, which is deemed promiscuous, and in her resistance to the roles held out for her. Kaysen is caught between these roles and some as yet undiscovered life or identity. Since this is unrealizable, Kaysen's only option is resistance, "negation," an option that also brings desolation and emptiness. Without a way to articulate her refusal of traditional feminine roles, and without a visible alternative, Kaysen is paralyzed, suspended in the "parallel universe."

Trauma and Shattered Subjectivities

In comparison to Kaysen's inward states of alienation and emptiness, many contemporary borderlines describe more debilitating, turbulent emotional lives and embodied stresses. They describe more profound feelings of self-hatred and depression, and express these feelings through attacks on their own bodies, including eating disorders and self-mutilation.

Jane Wanklin, in her 1997 autobiography *Let Me Make It Good*, describes the complicated picture of long-term disturbance that Irving Yalom confronts in his patient Marge: "multiple suicide attempts, eating disorder . . . episodic psychotic thinking, twenty-three years of therapy." In her narrative, Wanklin truly embodies the unlivable space of the abject feminine. She describes profound feelings of depression and self-loathing, coming repeatedly to her intense feelings of badness and worthlessness. Wanklin also recounts her repeated episodes of self-mutilation, which often precipitate her many psychiatric hospitalizations. Her narrative reflects the "angry, self-damaging" actions captured by the post-1980 descriptive definition of borderline personality disorder found in the DSM-III and IV.

According to Judith Herman, the many and varied symptoms associated with borderline personality disorder have their origin in a history of childhood abuse. She states that "The earlier the onset of abuse and the greater the severity, the greater the likelihood that the survivor would develop symptoms of borderline personality" (Herman 1992, 126). Herman points out that survivors of abuse present a "bewildering array of symptoms" and have higher levels of distress than other patients. She cites the findings of one psychologist who reports that survivors of childhood abuse "display significantly more insomnia, sexual dysfunction, dissociation, anger, suicidality, self-mutilation, drug addiction and alcoholism than other patients" (122–123).

Jane Wanklin, with her multiple symptoms of severe anorexia and bulimia, panic attacks, depression, self-mutilation, and drug and alcohol abuse, would appear to fit Herman's profile of a survivor of childhood abuse. Yet unlike many borderline patients, Wanklin describes a stable and even loving early family life, with no parental abuse. The stresses in her life, rather, appear to be located in the outside society, in the disillusionment of the post-1960s culture with its political assassinations, failed acid trips and drug exhaustion, escalating sexual violence, and burgeoning 1970s media culture. Jane Wanklin struggles through the contradictory pressures of drugs, sex, ultrathinness, and high achievement expected of young, privileged white girls in the 1970s and 1980s. Her emaciated, scarred body becomes the sign of burn-out and of the long-term institutionalization that her life becomes by the mid 1990s.

However, early childhood trauma will emerge in the narrative in the form of a recovered memory from Wanklin's infancy, and will provide the singular answer to the mysteries of her multiple disturbances. The trajectory of the narrative moves toward the revelation of the secret of repressed memories of abuse, and its recovery provides the resolution to the tension of Jane's escalating psychological pain. Thus, the narrative structure of Wanklin's autobiography resembles that of the case history in its search for origins. The discovery of the origin of symptoms is privileged in the case history, and, according to Peter Brooks, this is what gives it its narrative authority. "The authority of narrative derives from its capacity to speak of origins in relation to endpoints" (Brooks 1984, 276). The revelation of the abuse is the climax both of Wanklin's illness and of her narrative.

Yet while Judith Herman's analysis provides a framework for understanding the origin of Wanklin's symptoms, particularly her self-mutilation, as a response to abuse, Wanklin's symptoms appear to be overdetermined, with multiple sources rooted in her response to the contradictions and pressures of gender subjectivity in society.

Wanklin's account opens in the context of the social turmoil of the late 1960s. Wanklin situates her sense of placelessness and depersonalization in the events of this sociopolitical terrain. She reacted strongly to the assassinations of Robert F. Kennedy and Martin Luther King, Jr. She explicitly connects her first experience with depression to the assassination of Robert Kennedy, saying to a friend, "'Now I know there's no hope for this world we're living in. . . . I can't see growing up in a place where good people keep getting blown away like this.' When Kennedy died, just like his brother five years before, I suffered my first really deep depression and wouldn't emerge for a very long time" (20).

In 1967, she writes, she was introduced to "the Vietnam war, the growing drug problem and the gradual disillusionment of youth for the society in which it was forced to exist. . . . Even our music seemed to be acquiring a cynical, bitter edge, one that alternately repulsed and intrigued us" (19). Her response is depression, which escalates in the confusions of adolescence. Jane sees herself caught not only on the border between childhood and adulthood, but between a more innocent society and a newer world of drugs, permissive sexuality, and political turmoil. In the midst of what she calls the "psychedelic vacuum" of 1970s, she escapes into the world of 1950s music. "I remember wishing fervently that Time would magically begin a period of reversal to a more freshly scrubbed and musically pure state. I knew, realistically, that this was futile dreaming" (57).

She sees herself as a "true enigma": "a displaced child who refused to grow up and enter a new, frightening decade, one that was heralded in with the four student shootings at Kent State University in 1970. I despised the world in which I was living and the way it was affecting everyone. There had to be an effective way of staving it off" (30).

Her strategy for staving off the turbulence of adulthood is anorexia. At war with her body, she succumbs to an extreme disdain of her body and fear at her hunger. Her first crisis happens at the age of sixteen, when she begins what will become a lifelong struggle with anorexia and exercise obsession. Comparing herself to models, television stars, and other girls in her high school who have successfully dieted, she strives to attain a "sylph like" body. "Nothing, I vowed, summing up every fiber of stubbornness in my tortured teenage soul, would stop me from achieving this stellar goal" (33). She begins starving herself. She illustrates her sense of herself as nothing without that sylphlike body, and the feeling that all her value and worthiness lie in her achievement of this body. She turns herself into a "shadow girl," in her words. Thinness has become her regulatory ideal, her sole identity. As Bordo's analysis of anorexia illustrates, the disciplinary regimen of starvation and exercise embodies Foucault's conception of "power from below" when the subject actively strives to attain normalization through discipline of the body (Bordo 1993). The anorexic embodies the split in Western culture between mind and body, with mind striving to master and discipline the unruly appetites and contours of the body. The paradox of anorexia, of course, is that the harsh discipline required begins to control the mind. For Wanklin, "a horrifying transformation began to take place. I was no longer controlling the diet; it was slowly and cruelly manipulating me. It wasn't a matter of choice anymore, but one of urgent necessity. A new, disturbing element was added to the bizarre mixture: Fear. It propelled my dwindling body into wild spasms of exercise to such an alarming extent that my physical movements became focused and exaggerated" (Wanklin 1997, 36).

Wanklin's account also illustrates the gendered quality of the split between mind and body, in her explicitly seeking to lose weight to win her father's approval and love. "Though I wasn't actually overweight, and never had been, I was what my father termed 'chunky' (a word I grew to despise). I knew at a very young age that my father preferred skinny women. . . . As a doleful adolescent who desperately craved Daddy's affection, I wondered then that if I was really thin, he'd pay more attention to me. That's how young girls' minds work; I was nothing unique" (33). When her dieting turns excessive and she begins starving herself, going down to eighty-seven pounds, she imagines that her father is pleased. Food is the enemy, and she fears it will make her "ugly again, and no longer the center of my father's attention" (51).

Wanklin is initially rewarded for her self-denial, with other high school classmates showering her with compliments. Yet her social acceptance is short-lived as she discovers that her world has narrowed to the tunnel vision of calorie counting and obsessive exercise. She fails to make cheerleading or team sports, and she remains socially isolated. She continues self-starvation and is hospitalized for six weeks.

In addition to craving her father's attention, Jane views her feelings of worthlessness as rooted in her "lifelong belief that my parents loved my brother more" (61). As a result, she identifies with males and even wishes she were a boy. "So intense was my conviction that I'd really wanted to be a boy," she writes, that she "searched for a reflection of myself in all the boys and men of the media that I adored" (61).

But more than about gender confusion, she also worries about her sexuality. She describes her "growing sense of confusion about her sexuality" and wonders why she lacks interest in "guys." Yet in the midst of compulsory heterosexuality and homophobia of the late 1970s, and with no place to express such feelings, she is herself confused and shamed by her feelings.

Determined to seek out male attention, Wanklin finds that heterosexuality is fraught with dangers. During high school, she has what she refers to as her "head-on collision with heterosexual sex and mind-altering drugs," thus plunging her into the dangerous world she has attempted to stave off. In her longing to be part of a group of "cool kids" she begins spending time with an acquaintance who has his own apartment. She begins taking drugs and meets Wayne, who becomes her boyfriend. She takes acid with Wayne and his crowd. She vividly describes her harrowing response to the acid, as she erupts in panic and sobs uncontrollably. Not long after this, Wayne, who has been pressuring her to have sex, finally forces himself on her. Caught between the fears of appearing to be an "immature baby" and her terror, she faces not only the pain of the rape, but the denigration of Wayne's friends when they find out. They treat her with contempt, calling her a "slut" (73). Jane views these events as "the death of my childhood dreams" (73).

Wanklin's experiences with sex in high school only reinforce her self-loathing. Later in college, after she has unprotected sex with Burton, she fears she may be pregnant. When Burton leaves her for another girl, she writes, "I was very upset and felt the pain clear into my hair follicles. I had been dumped, in favor of a better, more wholesome girl, just as I had by Charles and Simon. I must be some kind of repulsive freak, I thought. I truly hated myself" (112).

Wanklin encounters similar dangers from some of her therapists. When Jane's parents arrange for her to see a therapist to help her in the midst of her anorexia, he tells her that she "desperately craved love and affection from a dominant male personality" and begins a personal relationship with her. He writes her poetry and conducts their therapy sessions at his apartment. His personal attention culminates one day in an attempt to have sex with her. Wanklin escapes, infuriated. "I felt embarrassed, humiliated and betrayed. How could a man who wrote such insightful and sensitive poetry be such a lech?" (55) She has a similar encounter several years later while in college. She seeks help for depression from a psychologist who, she writes, "turned out to be another lecherous shrink" who tells her all she needs is sex (118).

During her first year at college, a gay male friend tells her, "It sounds as if you might be bisexual," and introduces her to his lesbian friends, who take her to a lesbian bar. She is picked up there, but is not able to allow herself to go beyond a good-night kiss. "My conscience, formed by many years of a fairly religious upbringing, as well as a hefty dose of moral hypocrisy, dictated that it was wrong to love someone of the same sex. It would only bring shame and retribution upon me and my family" (95). She is drawn to a gay identity, but her guilt overrides her desires. She resolves never to return to the bar.

Wanklin's feelings of worthlessness and shame coalesce in her repeated episodes of self-mutilation. The theme of self-mutilation is hinted at in the opening chapter, when she describes feeling fascinated, at the age of four, with the sight of her mother's hot iron, and quickly places a finger on it. After the first agony of physical pain has passed, she notices something "oddly positive" about the pain. "It distracted me from the constant, dull ache that was ever present. It wasn't really a hurt, but more of a sadness" (4).

Later, at age seventeen, she cuts her forearms with a razor blade, to escape her constant psychic pain. She cuts a gash in her arm, then cuts horizontally across the cut, forming a cross. "Mentally, I felt better, less distraught, as I let the pain sink me in a warm release" (78).

What Wanklin is describing is echoed in the experiences of many others who self-cut. Self-cutting, writes Marilee Strong, can be understood as an attempt to make tangible and concrete a psychological pain, and thereby dispel profound feelings of badness and emptiness. It is, in the words of one of her interviewees, a "bright red scream," a "graphic cry for help" (Strong 1998, xviii). One of the women Strong interviewed, Josie, describes her cutting as a way of managing her pain: "I feel I have to control or contain the rage or whatever emotion is overwhelming me, and hurting does that. Cutting substitutes the pain inside with a physical pain that I can control, which is easier to handle. The pain is now real, tangible. It can be seen" (43).

Wanklin's self-cutting emerges again during college, when she is enveloped by deep depression. Her parents' marriage, long failing, has ended, and she is saddened by the "death of our family" (Wanklin 1997, 111). She has difficulty concentrating in her classes and begins to abuse alcohol. After another hostile rejection from a potential boyfriend, to whom she had written a passionate love letter, her feelings of self-hatred and depression escalate. She seeks help from a psychiatrist, who prescribes Librium and Anafranil, an antidepressant. Several days later, profoundly depressed and intoxicated, she attempts suicide by swallowing a handful of Librium. She is interrupted by her roommate, who calls Wanklin's father. Thinking she has simply drunk too much, her father sits with her while she sleeps. For her, the event is a turning point. "After that night, nothing was the same again" (118).

Her self-cutting is precipitated by a professor's accusation of plagiarism. Devastated, she gets drunk while listening to music. The voices singing in her speaker, which had provided a means of identification and comfort, turn on her: "Suddenly, frighteningly, a strange, sinister voice began taunting me from my left stereo speaker. I had been experiencing a lot of these auditory phenomena lately but none of the voices had sounded negative before. It was a male voice, low and evil-sounding, and began chanting repeatedly, in a throaty, flat tone, 'You know what you have to do. Punishment is in order'" (125).

She had purchased razor blades the day before, and is now convinced that she should end her life. She cuts a slash across her wrist, but is discovered by her roommate. She is admitted to the psychiatric wing of the local hospital.

Thus begins a series of repeated hospital stays, and escalating episodes of rage and self-mutilation. The account revolves around her repeated episodes of self-cutting and psychiatric hospitalization, in cycles of escalating tension, dysphoria, and rage, followed by cutting, discovery of her act, and hospitalization or chemical or physical restraint.

She is transferred to a psychiatric facility and prescribed antipsychotic medication, which causes severe, debilitating side effects. She begins to experience terrifying periods when her eyes spasmodically roll to the side and freeze in that position. She is unable to control these movements, but the staff believes she is doing it deliberately. When she has convulsions and seizures, the staff responds by putting her in seclusion. She later learns that eye spasms are the result of a reaction to her medication (184). Yet doctors interpret her reactions as "acting out," thus perpetuating a cycle of misunderstanding that binds her ever more firmly to the identity of mental patient.

In the midst of grappling with the effects of medication, Wanklin still has the urge to self-cut. Shortly after being admitted to the psychiatric facility, she hears the voice again, instructing her to cut herself. Caught by a staff member, she is given a shot of Thorazine. Feeling numb from the medication, she panics at sensations of nothingness (133).

Her feelings of numbness cause her to view her body as strange and alien, and her anorexia returns. In one vivid passage, her distorted body image and her urge to cut herself come together: "This intense self-loathing caused me to appear swollen and hideous to my own senses. I would lie in bed and run my hands over my body, touching great, shuddering rolls of flab where, in reality, there were only bones. I wanted to take a sharp object and hack the imaginary adipose tissue from my frame, exposing beauty and virtue. Then, perhaps, the tremendous guilt would disappear, or at least lessen in intensity" (144).

This passage illustrates the fact that Wanklin, through her desire to erase her flesh or to cut it, is at war with her body. One part of her condemns her body; she loathes the part of her that is weak, deficient, and her self-loathing takes the form of an internal voice. The presence of critical, judgmental voices is commonly associated with both self-cutting and eating disorders. Fiona, a woman suffering from severe anorexia and self-mutilation who is interviewed in Marilee Strong's book on self-mutilation, A Bright Red Scream, describes the internal voices she hears: "You know they're not real. But it's like you're battling a subconscious that is speaking to you louder than you can talk. It could be the voices of people you know, people who have put you down, saying, 'You're horrible, you're ugly, you're fat.' Or it could be your own voice" (Strong 1998, 115).

Fiona's and Wanklin's voices, rather than a sign of schizophrenia, could be interpreted as the internalization of society's denigration of women; the voice of what John Berger called the "Surveyor," as Elaine Showalter says: "the running critique of appearance and performance that the woman has grown up with as a part of her stream of consciousness" (Showalter 1985, 213). An internalized part of the self, it is nonetheless split off and takes on a separate existence, frequently, as in Wanklin's case, taking the form of a male voice.

Significantly, studies have shown that anorexia and self-mutilation often appear together. Marilee Strong reports that "from 35 to 80 percent of cutters also suffer from eating disorders" (Strong 1998, 116). Strong found that roughly 80 percent of the people she interviewed had significant problems with food.

What appears to link eating disorders and self-cutting is a common origin in trauma.

> The fact that cutting and eating disorders often coexist should not surprise us, as the two behaviors share many of the same roots and serve many of the same functions. Both syndromes are frequently driven by trauma, especially sexual abuse, and can serve as ways to symbolically reenact the trauma while exerting some control over the situation. Each uses the body to work out psychological conflicts, to obtain relief from overwhelming feelings of tension, anger, loneliness, emptiness, and self-hatred. . . . And they each involve attacks on the body, a disturbance in body image, and an attempt to control body boundaries. (117)

Paige, a woman interviewed by Cauwels who had been diagnosed as borderline but who believes she has post-traumatic stress disorder, describes her hatred and denial of her body in response to sexual abuse to her mother's stringent control of her eating. Paige describes being abused by a neighbor from ages two to ten, with the abuse necessitating trips to the hospital for urinary tract infections and lacerations. In addition, she was sexually abused by her father. Her mother monitored everything Paige ate, even taking her to Weight Watchers at the age of seven. "Anything was more normal to me than eating. Between what was being poked into my body at one end and what I wasn't allowed to put into my mouth—and later, to be put on a drug that made me fat, so that the psychiatrist who kept increasing the dosage put me on a diet . . . to this day, if I could be anything, I would be a floating mind. Get rid of this package—that would be the ideal state for me" (Paige, in Cauwels 1992, 88).

Unspeakable Acts and Embodied Memories

Scars are stories, history written on the body. (Kathryn Harrison, in Strong 1998, 17)

For those who have suffered early childhood trauma, the memory of the abuse is frequently split off and repressed, and yet may be encoded and enacted through the body. Traumatized people, Judith

Herman writes, "relive the event as though it were continually recurring in the present. They cannot resume the normal course of their lives, for the trauma repeatedly interrupts. It is as if time stops at the moment of trauma" (Herman 1992, 37). Time is frozen, and they relive the event, not through conscious memory, but through a form of embodied memory: "The traumatic moment becomes encoded in an abnormal form of memory, which breaks spontaneously into consciousness, both as flashbacks during waking states and as traumatic nightmares during sleep" (37). Further, such embodied memories do not take a linear narrative form: "They are not encoded like the ordinary memories of adults in a verbal, linear narrative that is assimilated into an ongoing life story." Instead, they emerge in fragments of images and sensations, intruding on the individual's consciousness. These "intrusions" take the form of "active memory" in which the survivor of trauma reenacts the trauma repeatedly. Herman notes, "Even when they are not dangerous, they have a driven, tenacious quality. Freud named this recurrent intrusion of the traumatic experience the 'repetition compulsion'" (Herman 1992, 41).

Jane Wanklin's narrative describes her embodiment of traumatic narratives through her repeated rituals of self-cutting. Again and again, she describes feelings of desperation and the wish to die, and tells how she seeks relief in cutting or burning her hands or arms.

Yet the fear, pain, and rage associated with the trauma may be buffeted by an altered or numbed state of consciousness that serves to distance the person from the traumatic moment, resulting in psychic constriction: a feeling of inner deadness and alienation. Judith Herman describes this state: "Events continue to register in awareness, but it is as though these events have been disconnected from their ordinary meanings. Perceptions may be numbed or distorted, with partial anesthesia or the loss of particular sensations. Time sense may be altered, often with a sense of slow motion, and the experience may lose its quality of ordinary reality. The person may feel as though the event is not happening to her, as though she is observing from outside her body, or as though the whole experience is a bad dream from which she will shortly awaken" (Herman 1992, 43).

Herman relies upon Pierre Janet's concept of "dissociation": the splitting off of traumatic memories so that they are separate from consciousness (43). Originating as a coping mechanism to buffet the pain of the trauma, it involves the separation of one's mind and body, so that the person feels they are watching the events take place from a point outside themselves. "Pain is anesthetized. The individual feels depersonalized, numb, unreal, outside oneself, a dispassionate observer, rather than an anguished participant" (Strong 1998, 38). Dissociation may be so extreme that separate personalities are formed, leading to multiple personality disorder.

Self-mutilation is one of the common responses to trauma. Childhood sexual abuse, in particular, is found among a large percentage of those who engage in self-cutting. Cutting or harming oneself is seen as a response to states of unbearable agitation and self-hatred, as well as feelings of numbness or depersonalization. "The mutilation continues until it produces a powerful feeling of calm and relief; physical pain is much preferable to the emotional pain that it replaces. As one survivor explains: 'I do it to prove I exist'" (Herman 1992, 109).

For Herman, trauma provides a narrative comprehensibility to the variety of symptoms expressed by women diagnosed as borderline. It provides meaning, a life story, a "plot," that provides the connections between earlier events and later ones. The work of healing involves transforming the dissociated embodied memory into a verbal narrative, by "reconstructing the story." The survivor is encouraged to tell the story of the trauma. "She tells it completely, in depth and in detail. This work of reconstruction actually transforms the traumatic memory, so that it can be integrated into the survivor's life story" (175).

From this perspective, Wanklin's narrative can be understood as an attempt to "reconstruct the story," to render comprehensible the traumas of abuse, mental illness, and hospitalization. Wanklin's narrative moves toward accounting for her profound depression and rage, and her self-mutilation. As her narrative progresses, trauma begins to emerge as the key plot line that will make sense of her bizarre symptoms. The trajectory of the narrative moves toward the breakthrough of her repressed memory of abuse. Her recovery of this memory will provide the resolution to the tension of her escalating psychological pain. Her self-loathing, rage, and self-mutilation are posed as mysteries, clues that have an origin, a first event that stands as the singular source of her madness. The climax of the narrative is Wanklin's recovery of this origin.

The issue of trauma emerges in Wanklin's story in the form of "intrusions" of memory, when she begins to have flashbacks and nightmares. It begins one day when, while tasting vinegar from a bite of salt-and-vinegar chips, she has a flashback of a woman's face and a sense of dread and fear. Haunted by the vision, and immersed in the stories of child abuse she has been hearing in her support group for self-cutters, she begins to piece together a series of recurring nightmares. In them, she is very young, and is propped up in a chair, crying, and a woman is feeding her something sour tasting while shouting at her to "shut up, or I'll give you something to cry about!" (Wanklin 1997, 295) Her vision of the woman's face makes her believe it is her mother in the nightmares, leaving her with the conviction that her mother had abused her when she was an infant. "After that moment of revelation, it was as though a door had been flung wide open into my consciousness" (295).

Her nightmares escalate into violent scenes of being attacked with sharp objects in her vagina, accompanied by images of the "round-faced woman, surrounded by bright flames as she laughed maniacally at me" (301). Wanklin's symptoms begin to recur with ferocity, as her anorexia returns and she turns suicidal. "Life had become unbearable, with the nightmares and thinking that my mother had tortured me as a baby. How could I keep going with that awful reality?" (305).

Back in the hospital, she feels something threatening to intrude on her consciousness: "It seemed that there was something horrific and ugly, waving at me tauntingly from a distance and daring me to approach and be violently strangled" (309). She falls into a deep, paralyzing depression.

Wanklin's condition worsens in the hospital, as she begins having attacks of rage, which she calls "The Beast." The Beast "spring[s] from" her, causing "angry, frenzied outbursts" that result in her being put in full ankle and wrist restraints. Her memories finally break into consciousness in a climactic scene with Marie, a nurse she has befriended, when she feels a "frantic storm" well up inside her in response to the image of the maniacal woman in her nightmares. Frightened, she screams, "Stop It! Stop laughing at me like that! Haven't you done enough to me?" Finally she bursts out, "I hate my mother! I hate what she did!" (313).

With this confession, the mystery has been solved with the revelation of the repressed memory of abuse: "It was out. The deadly, terrible secret I'd been pushing into the dark, murky recesses of my consciousness for so long now had been unleashed upon this loving, compassionate woman. Marie took me in her arms and held me while I sobbed loudly and brokenly, my tears drenching both of us" (313).

Yet her horror at the possibility that her mother could have abused her still torments her. She continues what she comes to call her "blood rituals," slashing her forearm so deeply that she needs eighteen stitches. She finally confronts her mother, and has "the ecstatic revelation that it hadn't been my mother after all who'd molested me as a baby" (330). Her mother confirms to Wanklin that she had hired a baby-sitter for Jane when she was twenty months old. Her mother also informs her that the baby-sitter had a history of psychiatric problems, leading Wanklin to conclude that it was the baby-sitter who had abused her.

What is significant about this revelation is how it affects Wanklin's psychological state. She believes all of her symptoms are related to this early event, and this conclusion enables her to improve: "I got much better after that, although I hadn't come to terms with the trauma that the troubled woman had brought into my life and how, thirty-eight years had been devastated and practically destroyed because of the things she did" (332). Feeling "tired of mutilating my body," Wanklin finally stops cutting herself, though she attributes this in part to a change in her antidepressant medication. She improves enough to be released from the hospital.

Viewed through the lens of Judith Herman's analysis of trauma and memory, Jane Wanklin's recovery of a traumatic event renders her symptoms meaningful as adaptive responses to an external event. From this perspective, her self-cutting and anorexia are understood as coping strategies, as ways of "reenacting the trauma while exerting some control over the situation" (Strong 1998, 117). These seemingly incomprehensible actions are thus made intelligible as responses to a past external event over which Wanklin had no control. Trauma thus provides a "reason" for her actions, as Herman's patient put it. It thus shifts the causative agent from Wanklin—or more precisely, Wanklin's underlying psychopathology—to a social situation. In doing so, it gives her symptoms a history.

Yet Wanklin's own narrative appears to complicate this early childhood interpretation as the sole cause of her conflicts. Her account includes the sociocultural and gendered landscape within which she constructs her subjectivity. Her narrative returns repeatedly to gender conflicts in her life and to her present secondary status as a woman— her feelings of inferiority and sense of secondary status in the family in comparison to her brother; her awkward need for her father's approval, particularly of her outward appearance; her account of being raped in college; unwanted sexual attention from therapists; and devaluation by other men who have rejected her. Jane Wanklin is defined, and defines herself, as the object of male evaluation and attention. She has internalized her oppression, and feels her only worth or value lies in her outward appearance, reducing her identity to that of a body-object. Further, she has internalized the devaluation of femininity in her self-loathing, particularly of her own sexuality.

At the same time, her conflicts must be understood in the context of the turbulence of the decade of the sixties and seventies, the "psychedelic vacuum." Wanklin faces adolescence in a world that appears to have lost its innocent facade, marked in her account by the political assassinations of the Kennedys and Martin Luther King, Jr. The social changes of this period appear to offer newfound freedoms for women, but these appear threatening to her. The new sexual freedoms are fraught with danger and devaluation. While she is expected to excel academically, she also faces the ongoing pressures of being "beautiful and sophisticated," which for Wanklin means being exceedingly thin. She is steeped in media images and messages which reinforce her conformity. She is expected to use drugs to fit in, and does so to be accepted rather than for her own pleasure. Like Jane Flax's patient Laurie, Jane Wanklin faces contradictory and confusing expectations that, while seeming to offer more freedom and opportunities for women, nonetheless require conformity to outward images of feminine appearance, at the same time suppressing women's autonomy and sexual agency. Hence, given the complex social circumstances, Wanklin's symptoms can be understood to be overdetermined, not traceable to any single cause, but rather, the product of the variegated elements of a patriarchal culture.

Wanklin is determined to discover the past childhood origins of present psychological disturbances, and her narrative shares some significant features with those of the psychotherapists. She searches for a singular individual cause, in early childhood, of the complexities of her symptoms. Thus, like the psychotherapeutic narrative, Wanklin's tends to reduce the multiple social and discursive elements that may contribute to the forms and severity of her psychological responses. While Kaysen directly challenges the conventions of feminine normality against which she is defined as borderline and thereby makes connections between social definitions of feminine identity and her own psychic alienation, Wanklin does not make this connection directly. These complexities, however, are apparent in her account.

Conclusion

As the cases discussed show, the depiction of borderline patients by therapists captures the complexity of the subjectivities of borderline patients. Their analyses reveal the division in these women's psyches that fragments their subjectivities into a surface persona and an inner one that is split off in a realm of repressed desire, emotion, and memory.

Stein sees the symbolic significance of Ms. V.'s rituals of making up her "faces" and connects her need for an outward face to the wearing of a mask. His associations to her rituals lead to his recognition of her sense of deep shame and self-loathing, and her sense of invisibility and nothingness without the outward mask.

Yalom, too, recognizes in his patient Ginny the conflict between the "hostess parts of herself," the part that is oriented toward pleasing others, and her "true self"—the self with rage, greed, self-assertiveness, and personal desire. Listening to her in therapy, he hears the voice of the inner critic, the "pleasure-stripping voice" that suppresses her desires.

In his later narrative of his patient Marge, Yalom not only hears, but sees this suppressed, desiring self when Marge's alter-self, Me, breaks through her passivity. Yet in his evocative rendering of this double, Yalom constructs Me as a powerful seductive feminine image, one he will, as he writes, "sacrifice to the goal of integrating Marge's self" (Yalom 1989, 226).

While therapists rely on the dominant narratives of pre-oedipal selfhood to understand their patients' psychic fragmentation as "developmental deficits" (that is, Ms. V. is caught in a need to punish her introjected "bad mother"; Ginny's orientation toward others, according to Yalom, is a holdover from infancy), the fragmented and oscillating subjectivities described in these narratives can be read as intelligible responses to divisions in the cultural construction of gender. The borderline woman's split self embodies, in exaggerated form, the irreconcilable images of women in Western perception: that of the passive, dependent object of others' expectations, and the powerful autonomous position of active, desiring subject. Marge's crisis of identity is expressed as a split between a passive, dependent, powerless persona and an empowered, yet forbidden double. Laurie, too, as Flax shows, appears to be responding to the contradictory demands of a socially sanctioned feminine selfhood and a forbidden autonomy and empowerment. Laurie suppresses her rage and desire because these are culturally forbidden for women in Western society. Meanwhile, her outer conformity meets the social expectations of femininity as other-oriented, passive, and reflective of men's needs and desires. This fragmentation and oscillation between these two modes of being can be characterized not as pathological instability, but as a fluctuation between subject positions. The cultural construction of women as Other makes this figure of autonomous and powerful womanhood all the more threatening both to the analyst and to the patients themselves. Yalom's vivid portrait of this powerful woman reduces the threat by sexualizing and finally sacrificing her.

The autobiographical narratives provide a means of seeing how the double bind of women's identity affects their self-concepts, and how they come to understand and narrativize their subjective distress. Kaysen resists performing the socially condoned feminine roles that are held out for her. Caught between her resistance and her inarticulate desires (for love, for writing), she seems frozen in suspended animation, in a paralysis that brings with it emptiness, alienation, and desolation. It is only later, when she is able to connect to and realize her desires by finding a subjective place for a life of writing, that she is healed.

Jane Wanklin describes a more extreme fragmentation. She is at war with herself, exacting harsh discipline over her hunger in her anorexia, and fighting against a constant impulse toward self-destruction. Wanklin, like Ms. V., Laurie, and Ginny Elkin, has been striving to meet the social expectations of femininity, yet in extreme and graphic ways. She internalizes the denigration of women who violate these norms, punishing herself over and over for failing to attain the worthiness that she imagines is embodied in the regulatory ideals of feminine body and self. The pressure of these ideals is exacerbated in the post-1960s media culture of commodification and consumption in which she becomes enveloped.

Wanklin's recovery of a repressed memory of abuse alters the meaning of her symptoms, transforming them from the seemingly meaningless eruptions of an underlying psychopathology, to responses to an external situation over which she has no control. Wanklin relies on the narrative power of a single origin that provides the answers to her distress. Yet her own narrative shows her grappling with a particularly stressful and disempowering social world. Her sexual abuse might be viewed as an extreme form of the power that suppresses women's autonomy and leads to dissociation and to women's extreme attempts to gain control of their bodies.

For these women, shedding the dependent passive feminine self is more than a matter of individual adjustment; since it is a position structured into the logic of gender within which they construct their identities, they cannot step outside these gender relations to reconstruct their identities. In addition, to enter the realm of the subject, the realm that formerly excluded them, women must disavow their feminine embodied qualities, which are viewed as threatening or dangerous in Yalom's words ("lethal" to Marge's "central" self).

Thus, women who come to be diagnosed as borderline can be said to be expressing in exaggerated form some of the effects of the very conditions for women's construction of self in late modern society; these symptoms are thus readable as the embodiments or literal inscriptions of the contemporary construction of gender.

Chapter 5	The "Fatal Attraction Illness"

Women and Borderline Rage

BORDERLINE WOMEN ARE positioned in the territory where identity is blurred and unstable. This borderland territory is a place of struggle over meanings. In my analysis of the theme of the borderline patient's blurred, fragmented, or oscillating self, and of the formal psychoanalytic interpretation and textual depiction of the borderline's unstable self, I drew on the feminist analysis of gender and subjectivity as a perspective from which to view this psychic instability in a sociocultural context, as a response to women's position at cultural borders.

In this chapter I discuss another response of inhabiting the borderland: active struggle or resistance. Borders are the site of strife, conflict, battles over where the lines are drawn. Borders require a "border machine . . . with its border patrol agents, secondary inspection, helicopters" (Hicks 1991, xxvi) to enforce an unnatural border against the resistive efforts to redefine its location. These power struggles may be bloody and violent.

"Struggle" or "battle" may be accurate words to describe the way the therapeutic relationship with borderline patients is described in the cases analyzed in this chapter. A central theme in these cases is the anger of the borderline patient, an anger that destabilizes the therapeutic relationship and interrupts the work of therapy. In the case narratives, this uncontrollable anger is frequently described as rage.

"Rage" is a significant term. The word "rage" implies anger that is out of control, out of proportion to the situation, and therefore without reason.

In his linguistic analysis of anger, George Lakoff states that its many metaphorical connotations are based on a folk theory of anger as heat that is building up pressure inside the body. Lakoff notes that one of the central variations on this metaphor is the metaphor of anger as fluid (Lakoff 1987, 383). Since there is an upper limit to the pressure that can build inside a body, anger is also conceived of as having a limit. When that limit is reached, anger erupts from the body: "We can only bear so much anger before we explode, that is lose control" (386).

Rage thus suggests the eruption of emotion that has been held back behind a barrier and has been allowed to grow in intensity and force. It is anger that has crossed the threshold of normality or reason, and is therefore transgressive, out of control. Rage is therefore a word that connotes the fury of madness; its Latin root is *rabies*, or madness.

This chapter discusses the psychiatric construction of this "borderline rage." I analyze two cases in which the borderline patient's anger is interpreted as a sign of an underlying disease or illness. I explore the devices used in the case texts on borderline patients to accomplish this medicalization of anger and its effects in the text, which succeed in masking or deflecting one possible source of women's anger: their subordinate position in a patriarchal culture. I focus on two central narrative devices that analysts use and that depoliticize women's rage: 1) the rhetoric of rage as a natural force or flood, in which psychiatrists use this metaphor to depict rage as an overwhelming, irrational force that is fundamentally separate from the borderline patient's self; and 2) a displacement of rage from paternal to maternal sources, in which psychiatrists attribute the sources of rage to early mothering while ignoring its sources in women's social relations in patriarchal culture. These rhetorical strategies renders women's rage pathological and medical, thus eliding their political meaning.

The "Fatal Attraction Illness"

An image of borderline personality disorder that has emerged in mental health discourse is that it is, as Janice Cauwels writes, "the Fatal Attraction illness. . . . Like its thematic predecessor, *Play Misty for Me*, the film *Fatal Attraction* presents examples of borderline behavior" (Cauwels 1992, 124). Both films, asserts Cauwels, portray female characters who have been rejected by their male lovers and respond to this rejection through rage and revenge. As the "other woman," the female protagonist has only a marginal position in her lover's life, and the drama of the film is her violent intrusion into his private, seemingly safe and orderly domestic sphere, where she threatens him and his family.

In a gesture that appears to make absolute the "traffic between cultural images and psychiatric ideologies" (Showalter 1985, 14), Hollywood film has been advocated as a valuable resource to teach mental health trainees and medical students about borderline personality disorder (Hyler and Schanzer 1997; Wedding and Boyd 1999). Steven Hyler and Bella Schanzer advocate the use of films such as *Play Misty for Me*, *Misery*, and *Basic Instinct* to teach students about various aspects of borderline personality disorder. But, they argue, *Fatal Attraction* is the best choice for "a single film that touches upon almost every aspect of the disorder" (467). "Alex Forrest's character is a superb portrayal of the psychological unraveling of the borderline personality. She goes to frantic lengths to prevent her lover, Dan Gallagher, from leaving her by slashing her wrists, hounding him, calling his home nonstop, and kidnapping his daughter for the afternoon. . . . Her impulsivity is demonstrated by the act of sleeping with a man she barely knows (criterion 4)." No mention is made of Dan's "impulsivity" in doing the same with a woman he barely knows.

In their 1999 book *Movies and Mental Illness: Using Films to Understand Psychopathology*, Danny Wedding and Mary Ann Boyd present a mock case report of the character of Alex Forrest, complete with psychosocial history, functional assessment, diagnosis, and treatment plan. In their typology of films, they call the Alex Forrest character the "femme fatale," and write that she is "a glamorous and sexually aggressive publishing executive" and that "the performance by [Glenn] Close dramatically illustrates many characteristics of patients with a borderline personality disorder: anger, impulsivity, emotional lability, fear of rejection and abandonment, inappropriate behavior, vacillation between adulation and disgust, and self-mutilation" (68).

Cauwels argues that both *Fatal Attraction* and *Play Misty for Me* are partially accurate in their portrayal of the borderline patient, but only, she states, "up to a point. The inaccuracy is that both films show the borderline character from her male lover's point of view, acting out the fury of the 'woman scorned'" (Cauwels 1992, 124). Missing, she argues, is a portrayal of the feelings that motivate the borderline to do the things she does. While Cauwels is concerned with going beyond the image to explore motivation, she nonetheless accepts the image itself as an accurate representation of the borderline woman.

This popular image is a troubling one, not because these uses of the film character of Alex Forrest portray her unfairly as "mad." Rather, what is particularly disturbing is that a fictive and misogynist cultural image of woman is presented as reality, and as an accurate picture of a woman with borderline personality disorder.

Alex Forrest is a single professional woman who initiates an affair with a married man. As Elaine Showalter observes, the female character represents women's sexual and professional freedom to "move in the public space of the city"; as the film progresses, this freedom is depicted in such a way that it "seemed to transgress male boundaries and endanger male sanctuaries" (Showalter 1990, 139). The film, writes Liahna Babener, emerged out of the conservatism of the late 1980s, and presents Alex Forrest as a "lone femme fatale preying on susceptible men for selfish ends. That figure of womanly evil is modernized in this Reagan era morality play, presented here as the self-advancing career woman Alex Forrest" (Babener 1992, 28). While the film begins with Dan Gallagher (portrayed by Michael Douglas) as guilty of an infidelity that threatens his family, "through adroit narrative, verbal and visual manipulation, responsibility for the catastrophe is shifted from male wrongdoing to female predation; what begins as a tale of a man's violation of the trust of his loved ones turns into a misogynistic rant against the social posture and sexual autonomy of the independent woman" (26).

The film accomplishes this by transforming Alex into a madwoman, thereby discrediting her demands. As Kathe Davis writes, "Most insidiously, Alex uses the catchphrases of the feminist movement to defend her indefensible actions. . . . She appropriates feminist positions, insisting on her right to recognition, reciprocity and respect and on shared male reproductive responsibility, couching her demands in feminist language. The complete illegitimacy of those demands in the context of the narrative serves then to discredit that language, as does her murderous insanity in general. . . . The maneuver is the age-old one of dismissing righteous female wrath as hysteria, and by ignoring it, transforming it into actual hysteria" (Davis 1992, 54).

Alex's climatic violent rage in the final scene is portrayed as her vengeful and hysterical, even psychotic, response to her rejection. Yet her vengeance provokes the fury of her lover, who wants only to be rid of her. The final scene of the film comes to a dramatic climax with Dan, as victim-turned-avenger, choking her to death in a murderous rage.

Thus, the autonomous woman loses out in the end, and the film's narrative climax is the violent rage targeted at her. The audience is encouraged to identify with Dan as victim; Alex, as the initiator of an illicit affair, is portrayed as lacking in moral grounding. Yet the effect, in the end, is the film's construction of the autonomous woman as threatened by and succumbing to madness, and the audience is encouraged to find her final annihilation justified. Showalter quotes Amy Taubin's comment in the *Village Voice* review of the film, that it recreates the patriarchal fantasy that the "sexually eager woman is just a gasp away from the castrating Medusa, the murderous phallic mother, and that if sex is not contained by marriage, it will be the end of civilization as we know it" (Showalter 1990, 139).

The depiction of the borderline personality as the "Fatal Attraction illness" thus suggests the image of the borderline as a powerful and destructive female figure whose irrational and violent rage victimizes men. While this image appears as a reductive, oversimplified stereotype, the image it portrays raises the question of the social links between this filmic construction of the vengeful raging woman and the psychiatric depiction of the borderline patient.

The Rhetoric of Rage

Rage is one of the central characteristics of the definition of borderline disorder. It is one of the symptoms of the borderline patient's instability of mood, and is thus one sign of the borderline patient's chaotic or oscillating selfhood.

In the case narratives, this uncontrollable anger is often described as a rage that has erupted or burst through the boundaries of the self. It is frequently described, like the symptom of emptiness, using metaphors of liquidity. The rage is described as a flood that swamps the borders of the self. Thus, women's anger in this psychiatric context is constructed as out of control and beyond the borders of reason, the mere primitive eruptions of a fragmented and unstable self.

This description of the borderline patient's anger as a flood is not confined, however, to psychiatrists; as the following example from a patient, Melanie, shows: "Borderlines have floods of emotions, as if a dam breaks. . . . When the emotions break loose, and they still do, it's like my total insides change. There's no way of stopping it. It's like a hemophiliac bleeding" (Cauwels 1992, 63).

The borderline patient's anger and hostility is a dominant theme in psychiatric discourse and marks the intensity of the relationship between patient and therapist. This anger has an unsettling effect on therapists. One psychiatric resident states, "Borderlines have a terrific anger. It's not only that the anger is powerful, but there's a certain quality to it. . . . I don't really have the words to describe it. . . . there's something disgusting about the anger. It's an unbearable anger" (quoted in Cauwels 1992, 27).

In the case narratives, the rage is often at the center of a struggle between analyst and patient, a battle of wills, language, and power. It is a rupture or disruption in the situation, and thus throws into question the analysis as well as the analyst's efficacy and authoritative position. It destabilizes the therapeutic relationship, causing intense countertransferential emotions in the analyst. Therapists may experience reactions of apathy, withdrawal, frustration, or may themselves experience anger, hostility, and rage at the patient. Nathan Schwartz-Salant writes: "The therapist attempts to buttress himself or herself against intense affects of hate, rage, hunger and envy, rather than voluntarily suffer them. Furthermore, he or she will often flee from the experience of chaos and from the pain of an absence of emotional contact with the patient" (Schwartz-Salant 1989, 7).

This rage may manifest itself as a negative or destructive energy, which is experienced as very powerful and unsettling to the analyst: As Schwartz-Salant writes, "Most upsetting is the expectation of being attacked, not by the patient's words but by an underlying, hateful energy that seems prompted by nothing less than the wish for the therapist's complete dissolution" (15).

The patient's rage may manifest itself more overtly as a resistance to the therapist, as a transgression by the patient of the norms of the analytic situation, or as a violation of the prescribed behavior of a "good" patient. Such intense struggle may account for the frequent description of the borderline patient's rage as toxic; it poisons the relationship and destroys any possibility for empathy by the therapist.

Therapists' reactions often plunge them into a state that resembles that of the borderline patient. As Theodore Nadelson writes, "The therapist is both the victim and the victimizer, dragged along in a sense of helplessness and frustration in a situation that mimics aspects of the patient's own life" (Nadelson 1977, 751). Schwartz-Salant says of therapists' reactions to the difficulty of the borderline patient, "The therapist has now become borderline! The patient is hated and treated without any sense of concern. . . . The patient is also defensively idealized as the therapist's hatred toward him or her is further split off through the ruse of deciding to be open, calm, and centered. Throughout, the therapist's self-hatred builds as a reaction to feeling so impotent and cowardly" (Schwartz-Salant 1989, 18).

Nadelson candidly expresses this sense of inefficacy: "When borderline patients accuse me of ineffectiveness, banality, or lack of understanding, I often experience discomfort accompanied by the conviction that the patient is quite correct. On one occasion, my thoughts ran as follows: 'I feel that I have not helped the patient, I am repetitious, perhaps I help no one.' There are times when I find myself wishing that I could stop treating such patients; I wish they would go away or die" (Nadelson 1977, 750).

This chapter discusses two cases in which anger figures prominently as a symptomatic sign of the borderline patient's unstable self: the case of Agnes, a nineteen-year-old patient analyzed by Manuel Ross, as presented in "The Borderline Diathesis" (Ross 1976) and the case of Mae, whose long-term psychotherapy with Richard Chessick is described in "Intensive Psychotherapy of a Borderline Patient" (Chessick 1982). In both cases, the patient manifests intense anger that is frequently directed at the therapist, and in both cases this anger is the central feature of the therapist's understanding of the patient's self as chaotic, unstable, or missing. This unstable self is traced to the unconscious emotional residue of the patient's archaic pre-oedipal relation with the mother. In attributing rage to the patients' prehistory—to their unconscious relationship with their mothers—these analysts fail to make connections to their patients' history—their biographical and social location. By "history" I mean not only specific biographical events, but also the position of borderline patients as women at this specific historical juncture, which has implications for patients' rage that go beyond the bounds of individual therapy but that nonetheless structure the analytic response and construction of this female rage.

The psychiatric construction of female rage as a prehistoric flood that has no sources other than archaic primitive ones perhaps satisfies an unconscious desire on the part of therapists to resolve the problem of the woman who overtly rejects her position.

The Hysteric as Borderline: Primitive Rage and the Missing Self

The case of Agnes illustrates the turbulence and intensity of the analyst's encounter with the borderline patient (Ross 1976). Agnes is a hospitalized borderline patient who is in treatment with Ross for almost four years. In his opening statement, Ross acknowledges the uncertainty in the meaning of the borderline label, and alludes to the use of the label as an answer to "perplexity and anxiety in the face of clinical data" (305). Furthermore, "we know that interpretation in the borderline and psychotic conditions is for long periods problematic if not impossible, unlike that of the neuroses (the unraveling of which Freud compared to the painstaking work of an archaeological dig where the forms of a previous civilization gradually come into view)" (305). After this acknowledgment, however, Ross then offers a definition: "In the borderline, as I hope to show, the difficulties lie not so much within the confines of the resistances engendered by an ego defending sequestered fixations, but more within the realm of the cohesiveness of the entire psychic organization or, to shorten it, the self" (306).

Ross, like many other analysts, defines the borderline patient as suffering from a lack of cohesive self; further, this lack of self is manifest in the patient's inability to offer a coherent narrative, which, for Ross, makes empathy between patient and analyst difficult or impossible. Commenting on the psychoanalytic process of interpreting the "undisrupted stream" of clinical data that the patient produces, Ross states that "the patient who has these areas intact communicates not only the pieces of data, but also the forms in which they are embedded so that we remember by large blocs in which each item falls into place automatically as it were, with minimal or no effort on the analyst's part. When it is working, as it does in the neurotic, it is subjectively felt as empathy, which is in itself an affective form based . . . on a successful interchange in the mother-child unit" (308).

The borderline patient lacks such narrative abilities. For the borderline, writes Ross, "the world is not timeless, but it is broken up into successive but unconnected bits. One hour does not lead to the next. Although this may be related to aggressive drives, the central defect is in the organizing structures of the self" (308). The borderline patient's narrative is incoherent; therefore, the self lacks an underlying structure. Ross's statement implies that it is not only the content of the story that lends it coherence, but its form or structure. Below the level of content of a patient's story, a certain structure is expected or the narrative is not a narrative; it lacks the minimum requirements of linear connection and logical flow of ideas. What is missing in the borderline patient's verbal productions, then, is not particular items of information, but the underlying narrative form.

To illustrate the borderline patient's incoherent narrative, Ross supplies a literary example. Ross draws parallels between the borderline's unconnected and incoherent narrative and modernist literature. For Ross, the only modernist author whose narrative structure resembles that of the borderline patient is Kafka. Kafka's works are without the kind of force and form that particular characters embody with their histories and their journeys that come to closure or finality. Kafka's "pure parable" without character history is a kind of borderline nonnarrative. For Ross, borderline patients are like Kafka's characters: "Kafka's description comes as close as any to describing the states of panic and estrangement in the borderline which so often precede acting out. It is the paradigm of estrangement. Yet, there is no break with reality, as in the psychotic, which paradoxically also means that there is no avenue for escape. It is this uncanny distress which helps to make the diagnosis of borderline pathology even if the phenomenology is diverse" (310).

Thus, the borderline patient manifests an "uncanny distress," a sense of estrangement, which, according to Ross's description, is expressed in an inability to communicate with others and hence a lack of empathy.

Ross notes that in spite of this "defect," which soon becomes evident to the analyst, the borderline patient appears not to be aware of it. The borderline patient, "having missed what Dostoevski has called the 'crucible of doubt' during development, appears intently certain. Indeed," Ross continues, "borderlines can be some of the most certain people in the world" (309). Here the contradictions in the meaning of the borderline diagnosis become apparent in the attribution of both incoherence and certainty to the same patient. In Ross's view, the borderline patient's instability is not an uncertainty or confusion—that is, an instability of which the patient would be aware, but rather a structural incoherence, evident to the observer but not to the patient. In psychoanalytic terminology, this is referred to as "ego syntonic"; these are psychological structures that are not troubling to the patient. Such a lack of self-awareness itself is viewed as evidence of a lack of ego control. The lack of ego boundaries clears the way for the eruption of unconscious forces.

Ross's patient Agnes manifests such lack of ego control, as well as the lack of a coherent narrative within the therapy hours. "From age 15 on, Agnes had led an increasingly disordered and aimless life characterized by promiscuity, drug usage and runaways. Her moods, which at first sight appeared unrelated to the observable events of her life, varied from prolonged sulking to states of rage which were run off at a howling pitch. She presented one emergency after another to the community and her pathology soon came to be a dominating element in her parents' life" (313).

The event that triggers her latest hospitalization is a suicide attempt. Prior to this, she was increasingly troubled by thoughts of suicide and had begun to burn her arms with cigarettes. She was eventually hospitalized for six months, and immediately upon returning home after being discharged from the hospital attempted suicide again by taking an overdose of barbiturates. It is this hospitalization that marks the beginning of her relationship with Dr. Ross.

One of the major qualities that Ross notices in Agnes is a lack of a self. During their first session together Ross notes that Agnes's narrative is fragmentary and incomplete: "In our first hour, Agnes cited some fragments of her history very intensely and it looked like she had a very firm idea of what she was talking about. . . . And yet, though each individual item seemed understandable in and of itself, little cohered together. . . . It was not emptiness, because that quality implied boundaries of the self. When I spoke to her at the end of the hours, I was not sure just whom I was addressing and I had an uncanny sensation of addressing a set of random facts rather than a self" (310).

Ross is also unable to obtain Agnes's narrative of her dreams. "I could not obtain a discrete dream text. . . . I could not tell where the dream left off and where her associations began" (316).

Agnes speaks to Ross of her own uncertainty and confusion, her inability to define herself and to define who her analyst is: "The issue was not content but the boundaries of that content. In one hour she became distraught and said, 'Who are you? Who am I? I want you to get inside me and rummage around and find out who I am.' There were a number of variations of this theme, some of them occurring much later in treatment. Invariably, the 'who am I?' brought with it the congener of 'who are you?'" (314).

While Agnes seems intangible to Ross at one level, at an emotional level she is unmistakably present. Agnes's rage becomes a dominating theme in Ross's narrative. "On the unit, Agnes showed much of what brought her to the hospital. She would have fits of rage. A number of times she collapsed to the floor and had what looked like attacks of colic as she clutched her abdomen and gasped for air" (314).

Her treatment with Ross settles into what Ross calls a "form of hostile relentlessness" that thwarts any attempt at psychotherapy. Ross comments, "I could identify no particular system of working through other than primitive discharge" (315). Ross depicts this "primitive discharge" as an uncontrolled forceful flow: "She was like a natural phenomenon and emotional responses to it would be like taking exception to the Niagara Falls." Ross's depiction of Agnes as a "set of random facts," or as emitting "primitive discharge," is here magnified in a metaphor that constructs the borderline patient as a "natural phenomenon" without agency, reason, or center—a blur. In this context, Agnes's rage seems, in Ross's view, the most tangible thing about her.

Further, with such a "primitive" psyche, Agnes is clearly marked off as borderline, at a "lower" level than the "neurotic": "For the most part, the doubt and curiosity that are shared in the analysis of a neurotic were mine and mine alone" (315). Agnes, unlike the neurotic patient, is not interested in or curious about her psyche or her analysis.

During the last year of their treatment, Agnes begins stealing, "a common symptom in borderlines," Ross notes (316). When she steals a pen from his office, he describes his intense countertransferential reactions: "At that moment I saw her as being utterly cannibalistic; everybody and everything, even the privacy of people she did not know, would have to submit to being drawn into the orbit of her pathology. At least with the pen, the issue was just between us. I found myself having a fantasy of pulverizing her hand by repeatedly jamming a heavy door against it" (316). This is a clear illustration of the intensity of countertransferential responses that the borderline patient incites in the psychiatrist.

To present his own analytic understanding of Agnes and similar patients, Ross draws on Freud's conflict with Dora (Ida Bauer), who, Ross feels, "suffered from something more than a neurosis" and whose work with Freud "resembled in outline the problems encountered with the contemporary borderline" (312).

> Nowhere else in Freud's work does one get such a trenchant picture of life in Vienna, with Dora contributing to this by her defensive emphasis on the external particulars of her life rather than on its more private vital core. Through complex sexual manipulations, there was a stultifying intrusiveness of one generation into another, Dora being both victim and the victimizer. It is not surprising that the analysis was caught up in this, especially in relationship to Dora's motivation for treatment. The termination was abrupt, which is not unusual in a borderline patient with the struggle to be avoided or not even conceived of. Perhaps, after all, she was unanalysable. Then there was the unnerving quality she had which left a deposit of uncertainty in Freud. There are a number of external indicators

of this, such as the misdating of the work (1899 instead of
1900—perhaps, after all, the work belonged more to the
nineteenth century), its delayed publication in the *Monatsschrift
für Psychiatrie und Neurologie* and Freud's shifting views about
where the work was to be placed. (312)

Ross also highlights many of the same elements of Freud's text that
feminist literary critics have analyzed: Freud's self-doubts, which reveal
the workings of countertransference in his interpretation of Dora. For
Ross, however, Freud's misgivings are evidence of Dora's having provoked him, and thus are evidence that she is borderline: "One can sense
that Dora had thrown Freud off stride, a common occurrence in the
work with the borderline where the position of receptivity in the analyst is repeatedly broken" (312).

Here Ross suggests that Freud's most famous case of a woman hysteric was in fact borderline. He states that Dora's narrative, like Agnes's,
is inadequate for analysis, because of her "defensive emphasis on the
external particulars of her life rather than on its more private vital core."
Ross is objecting to Dora's refusal to provide a story of herself, her narrative focusing instead on the people around her, the social network of
sexual exchange and complicity in which she is embedded. Dora's refusal or inability to tell the story of a private self becomes, for Ross, a
sign of her inherent character pathology. The statement about the "stul-
tifying intrusiveness of one generation into another, Dora being both
victim and the victimizer" (312) is curious, since it is left ambiguous
whether it is Dora or those of the other "generation" who are behind
the sexual manipulations and intrusiveness. Later Ross confirms his
judgment of Dora as the intrusive party, as he discovers in reading of
Felix Deutsch's rediscovery of and his interview with an older Ida Bauer
in "Footnote to Freud's Fragment of an Analysis of a Case of Hysteria"
(Deutsch, in Bernheimer and Kahane 1985). There, Deutsch writes that
Dora clung to her only son, and that "he often stayed out late at night
and she suspected that he had become interested in girls. She always
waited, listening, until he came home. This led her to talk about her
own frustrated love life and her frigidity" (37).

Ross writes, "She would await his return hoping to hear some signs
of frank sexual activity, having little sense of having a life of her own
except that which could be enjoyed vicariously from the scraps of some-

one else's excitement. Thus, Dora again was intruding into another generation, this time the younger one" (Ross 1976, 313).

Thus, Dora's positioning as an object of exchange in these familial social relations (her father's exchange with Herr K. in which Dora is traded for Herr K.'s wife) and her complicity in this arrangement, is here reduced to her character defect, which shows up in analysis as an inability to provide a coherent narrative of her "private vital core" of the self.

For Ross, Dora can be rediagnosed as borderline not only because she refused to provide a narrative of her self, but because of her overall effect on Freud. Ross notes that Dora had an "unnerving quality" that "left a deposit of uncertainty in Freud" (312).

Ross quotes Deustch's oft-quoted comment that one observer had called Dora "the most repulsive hysteric he had ever met" (313). Agnes is similar to Dora, Ross argues, because of the effect she has on him, "throwing him off stride." Agnes, like Dora, cannot provide a coherent self narrative. Thus, neither Agnes nor Dora before her has possessed selves.

For Ross, the trouble with Agnes's narrative is that it is infused with rage and appears outside any sort of narrative coherence. If Dora's narrative is piecemeal, relying on multiple bits of "gossip" and "external particulars," and is thus full of "holes" (Moi 1985), Agnes's narrative is disconnected from any social network, and thus does not have any sources at all aside from her own random outpourings. The problem for Ross is not ambiguity in Agnes's narrative, but the absence of any form of coherence in her person, so that he may surmise a self behind it. Ross confronts not so much a narrative with holes as a total lack—Agnes herself. Accordingly, he does not fill in the holes in Agnes's narrative so much as offer an explanation for the "hole" that is Agnes—a theory of her absence as a coherent self. He is thus able to provide narrative closure and totality to his text by describing what Agnes is not—empathic, coherent, and present.

It is from this perspective that Ross hears Agnes's rage. From Ross's object relations perspective, Agnes's rage and her lack of a distinct self are present manifestations of her state of arrested development in the pre-oedipal period, when the infant has not yet differentiated a self out of the fusion of the mother-infant bond. Thus, Agnes's rage is not so much composed of the tangible emotions of a perceptible personality as it is the expression of an isolated individual, disaffected and alienated. "It is not precisely hate, for hate implies an object and a conception of the self as relating to another self. . . . That is why I think estrangement is the better word to describe it" (Ross 1976, 317).

Ross roots Agnes's disorganized raging flood in the pre-oedipal period, when without a successful relation with the mother, profound estrangement is produced. Further, Ross anchors it to a biological source when he traces it back even earlier, to the patient's experience in the womb, writing, "The frequent history of drug usage in the borderline is related not so much to the oral period which is beset by rhythms, but more to the in-utero state where there is much neater biochemical mediation of distress" (311).

The important aspect of this case is the way in which the rage is connected to a missing self, which in turn arises from a unilinear conceptualization of the development of the self, in which the assumption is made that the more severe the pathology, the earlier in life its underlying causes are, and hence the more severe the self deficits will be. Thus the origin of borderline rage lies in the first three years of life.

Like Dora, Agnes terminates treatment: "Termination took place abruptly. She had missed two hours and was twenty minutes late for the session. She said right off, 'I decided to leave. I talked to Dad about coming home and he agrees. Don't give me any of your crap about thinking things over and I don't want to examine it. I've made up my mind.' The only thing I said during the hour was, 'This is a hell of a way to leave, but I suppose it's one way of doing it'" (317).

Ross's countertransferential feelings linger after her departure. "In the following four weeks I found myself relieved at not seeing her any more and even had the thought that I was now not seeing her intensively on a four-times-a-week basis. There was no doubt that she had left some wounds" (317). After receiving word from her father that she is "still having difficulties and that she now wanted to become a detective," Ross writes, "I thought how like Dora she had turned out, prying or at least having the fantasy of prying into someone else's life." Yet the following year the father writes that Agnes, now twenty-nine years old, shows no signs of her earlier difficulties and that her illness has disappeared as "miraculously as it had arisen" (317).

Ross confines his analysis of Agnes to the territory marked out by the object relational framework—the pre-oedipal sources of the patient's present behavior. Excluded from this framework and specifically from Ross's text on Agnes, is a consideration of her rage as intelligible—as a response to a particular event in her life, or to her social situation. Nothing appears in the text regarding Agnes's life or her history—which may have been the result of Ross's inability to obtain such a history, given the intense struggle between them. However, Ross does not refrain, even given the lack of information, from constructing an interpretation of Agnes. It is what she does not say, what she is missing—a coherent narrative—as well as her rage, that indicate to Ross she is borderline. Agnes's fury and resistance to Ross and to psychiatry are attributed to Agnes's prehistory, to the exclusion of her history.

Rage and Women's Resistance

In the case narrative featuring Mae, a borderline patient in long-term psychotherapy with Richard Chessick, this analytic displacement of rage and refusal onto the patient's prehistory is accomplished even when its sources in the patient's life are more visible and apparent (Chessick 1982). In this case, the patient's rage against representatives of patriarchal power—a theme highly relevant to an oedipal and therefore gendered interpretation—is displaced onto the pre-oedipal mother, the central figure in the object relations psychoanalytic framework. This case is therefore a good example of the limitations of the object relations account, specifically in excluding or distracting from the centrality of gender and power in women's construction of a self. The assumption that borderline disorder is pre-oedipal has specific effects in reproducing gender assumptions and minimizing the significance of the patient's rage.

In his account of the ten-year history of his treatment of Mae, Chessick summarizes the patient's state at the beginning of treatment as immature and undeveloped, the development and functioning of Mae's self having been thwarted by her "primitive rage." Chessick writes that "this report attempts to illustrate that 'deep' interpretations (for example, referring to the projection of split off self and object representations) early in the psychotherapy are ineffective, at least in cases such as this one. This, I believe, is primarily because that patient is not in a cognitive state or self state to utilize any interpretation, since the ego is occupied fully in dealing with the flood of affect—it is 'laboring badly'" (413).

As this quotation shows, Mae's rage is excluded by the analyst as a part of her self or ego. The rage is described as a "flood of affect," a primitive emotion that by definition, in the analyst's eyes, is "other" than her self, a "flood" that swamps any sort of selfhood. In place of a self, there are "primitive, unintegrated psychic structures" (415).

Mae saw Chessick from the age of twenty-six until she was thirty-six, from 1969 to 1979. Chessick at first describes her as "an attractive white woman of 26 years" and notes that she has recently terminated treatment by another analyst after only a few sessions. She is deeply resistant to the use of a couch during analysis, and sees it as intimately related to gender and power, placing her in a subordinate feminine position: "She stated that she absolutely did not want 'to lie down in front of a man' and that she had specifically been repeatedly warned by her mother never to do so. Mae described the couch as a 'torture instrument' and considered the situation, in which she could not see the therapist, as a form of intolerable deprivation, grossly unequal, and unfair" (413).

Thus the treatment begins with Mae's ambivalent relationship to therapy. On one hand, it is her current means of attempting to solve her problems, and on the other hand, she shows a resistance against filling the role of patient.

Mae also initiates treatment complaining of a lack of feeling or numbness—"frigidity" in Chessick's words—in relations with her husband. "After marriage she was disinterested in sexual relations and received no enjoyment from the sex act" (413). It is important to point out the significance of this opening to the narrative. The concept of "frigidity" defines dissatisfaction as a symptom. It is a concept that locates a problem of women's sexuality in the psyche and body of the patient rather than in her relations in the world. The patient, Mae, enters voluntarily into this framework of frigidity, by defining it as a problem to be solved by psychoanalysis, thus reproducing the assumption that the problem is located in her own mind, rather than in her social relations. Later in the narrative there is evidence of her dissatisfaction and anger at her husband's apparent lack of concern for her. Yet here it is defined as a psychogenic symptom.

Chessick points to the oddities in the patient's past history as evidence of a borderline condition underneath her presenting complaint of frigidity: "The history at first seemed to center around some hysterical problems, which probably accounted for the recommendation from the previous therapist for formal analysis. In spite of her careful control, however, there were some bizarre elements in the history that raised my suspicion of a borderline condition underneath the complaint of psychogenic frigidity" (414).

While Chessick goes on to discuss the patient's life history, he never specifies which particular elements warranted suspicion of a borderline condition, though he discusses several aspects of her childhood, such as the patient's having been raised in a strict Christian Scientist family: "Both parents were religious Christian Scientists and repeatedly made it clear that a child must fit the parent's mold, or something is dreadfully wrong and hellfire or sickness will result." Another biographical theme Chessick includes is Mae's parents' profession as funeral home directors: "She gave many memories of seeing her father cut open and embalm corpses and her mother paint their faces, comb the hair, and apply cosmetics to the dead" (414).

Mae's initial complaint of frigidity, Chessick soon discovers, gives way to an anger and frustration that seem to intensify with each session and further confirm the existence of a borderline condition: "The first six months of therapy were marked by an absolute flood of dreams that were often filled with rage and revolved around humiliation by men and devaluation of men. Also, she raged at the psychoanalyst, who she felt did not sense her hopelessness in the flood of all her hatred" (414).

Chessick several times in this selection refers to the "pouring out" of the patient's rage, which overwhelms her ego. This anger appears to threaten to overwhelm Chessick's relationship to Mae, and thus the therapy itself. He writes of his attempts to maintain his therapeutic stance: "The most important contribution that I made in this first year of the patient's treatment was to work calmly and relatively anxiety free, trying to understand this patient's material and not be sucked into the stormy chaos or panicked. Probably at the deepest level the main contribution I made was in not being destroyed by all her raging" (415).

Mae's rage, as Chessick writes, concerns men—including her husband, her father, and Chessick himself. At one point, Mae has an insight about her anger at men that involves her fear of them; "she actually preferred boys in high school and college who had problems with masculinity. Men who were vigorous thrusters frightened her because she saw the penis as a destructive weapon, so she was actually more comfortable with weak men" (416).

Her rage toward her husband centers on his preoccupation with himself and his apparent lack of concern for her. Mae's complaints about her husband frequently concern sexual issues. A key incident in the narrative is "her often-reported wedding night," when she awoke in the middle of the night to find her husband having sex with her. Chessick does not comment on this incident and presents it as yet another illustrative example of material that Mae presented in the therapy, which Chessick refers to as "complaints":

> Her sex life after marriage was extremely poor; her husband, who was the same age, seemed to have many problems about sexuality also. She described him as sensitive to others and loyal, but with a great need to succeed and prove himself a man. . . . He was described as a business executive who worked 70 hours a week in several jobs, but who got a promotion each time he moved from job to job. Their marriage was marked by extreme outbursts of rage on the part of the patient, which included throwing things at her husband; his only response was what she called a "sickly smile." (414)

In Chessick's narrative, material regarding Mae's husband is presented alongside material that arises regarding her father. "Whenever her husband came to her for sexual relations she was overwhelmed with rage and felt raped, attacked, and narcissistically used. Hatred of men was a continually dominant theme. Thus, she turned from her mother, who she said went vacuously through the motions of affection and care, to her father, who she spoke of as giving her 'tickling and teasing,' and a 'knuckle in the butt,' and 'embalming.' The penis was described as a 'hot glass' or a 'steel sharp cutter' and all sex as an ego trip for men" (416).

While in this segment and in the following one, Mae describes her mother as uninvolved and distant, she appears to present a more ambivalent association to her father and her husband, both of whom she likens to Chessick in the role of caretaker:

> Much of the second year was spent trying to reach a better adjustment with her husband, but she did not change and remained highly charged with rage and confusion. The patient accused both me and her husband of just going through the motions of playing our roles. She went on to relate how her cold and preoccupied mother went through the motions of taking care of her but used her for her narcissistic needs. She transferred her needs to her father, who would actually take her on his lap and be nice to her. But he had an enormous need to pinch her and tease her and scratch her with his whiskers, so that the patient continuously experienced the body warmth of a man along with painful sensations. (416)

Mae continues to have vivid associations of Chessick to her father. "Her reaction to my vacations remained unabatedly raging and unforgiving. Interpretations, as was previously described, did not help, and she responded by accusing me of teasing her like her father whenever I went on vacation. On several episodes she insisted that I looked exactly like her father" (416).

This mingling of the roles of father, doctor, and husband as targets of Mae's rage suggests her perception that they play a similar role in her life; that they have occupied positions of both caretaking and control, in legislating her emotions and identity. If she is to be a "normal adult woman," she will not complain about their control, but will remain passive. Yet her rage suggests her resistance against this stance.

Mixed in with Mae's rage in the therapy is her demand that Chessick meet her needs. She recognizes the "artificial barrier" between them that Chessick will not cross. She states that she holds a wish that she would be magically "fed" by Chessick:

> Gradually the rage shifted somewhat away from her husband and more and more on me, although the patient continued to be apparently devoted to treatment. She became increasingly sarcastic and hostile to me as she admittedly began to realize, already in the first year of treatment, that no massive "feeding"

(her term) or magical maternal giving was going to come from me. . . . The patient would rage at not being "fed," or she would progress to insisting that I could "feed" her but I malevolently refused to do it; at worst, she would say I demanded "feeding" off of her. . . . "Feeding," in her mind, was a code word for some sort of magical maternal giving and soothing. (415)

Chessick draws on the discourse of object relations theory to interpret Mae's demand or wish for "feeding" as a maternal demand, one rooted in the pre-oedipal relation to her mother. He states that her demands for "feeding" were signs of an "archaic self-object transference," that is, the unconscious transfer of past associations in her early pre-oedipal relation to her mother onto Chessick. Chessick's interpretation shifts away from the issues raised concerning Mae's relations with men, toward an earlier, more archaic relationship: that with her mother. This shift toward the importance of the pre-oedipal mother and away from the father is captured in a statement in which Chessick offers an interpretation of Mae's rage at men: "I believe that she was making all men into the bad mother and attempting to withdraw into a self-contained grandiosity. Similarly, in the transference I was experienced as the totally bad, unfeeling, narcissistically preoccupied, and unempathic mother" (416).

In the object relations interpretive framework, pre-oedipal dynamics are the focus. Mae puts Chessick in the role of "soothing self-object"—a pre-oedipal internalization of the mother. The patient is developmentally arrested in the stage of early "grandiosity," which, according to Heinz Kohut (1977), is rooted in early omnipotence characteristic of the condition of mother-infant fusion. In object relations theory, the narcissist clings to the illusion of omnipotence that precedes the gradual and more realistic awareness of the fallibilities of both the mother and the self. In later life, the patient comes to use these illusions of grandiosity as a defense against threats to the self posed by current relationships.

Hence, for Chessick, Mae's rage is "pathological." Mae's ego is "preoccupied with discharge of rage and fantasies of revenge," phrases that depict them as eruptions rooted in irrationality. Her rage is "exaggerated," based on paranoid feelings.

In addition to this understanding of Mae's resistance to therapy as "infantile," Chessick defines her rage as a force or flood that is outside the boundaries of her self. The rage has flooded and fragmented her sense of self. The separation of rage from the self effectively relegates the rage to a position outside the intelligible feelings or reactions of an adult. It is out of control—either childish, like a temper tantrum, or even inhuman, like Ross's "natural phenomenon," a force of "affect" that swamps the borders of Mae's self.

But the main interpretation of the rage, which is directly related to the main tenets of object relations theory, is Chessick's use of the conception of the "bad mother," so prominent in ego psychology and object relations theory, as both the original source of Mae's rage, and its ultimate (unconscious) target. Chessick traces Mae's conflict to "archaic" (that is, developmentally early) self and object representations. Thus, the ultimate target, and in effect, source of the rage, according to Chessick, is the "bad Omnipotent Mother" embedded as an archaic image, an object representation, within Mae's psyche. Though Mae manifestly rages at men, the true target of her rage is the pre-oedipal mother, toward whom she feels repressed rage at being deprived of gratification. Chessick's interpretive and textual displacement of rage at men onto the pre-oedipal mother is summed up in Chessick's conclusion that Mae is "making all men the bad mother" (416).

According to Chessick, Mae has been developmentally arrested at the early stages of ego development when the child feels omnipotent and grandiose, and attempts to magically control the environment, including the mother, to meet her narcissistic needs. Mae's demands that Chessick soothe, hold, and feed her are the demands of an infant on Chessick, who has posed, or refused to pose, as the fantasized pre-oedipal mother.

This fairly common interpretation of borderline disorder, when applied to Mae's rage at her powerlessness in gender relations, has the specific effect in this particular text of deflecting attention from another prominent source of her rage—the men in her life, as representatives of patriarchal power. The outcome of this displacement is the way the text masks, or turns the reader's attention away from, that patriarchal power itself as an equally viable target of Mae's borderline rage.

Chessick demonstrates an awareness of these other sources of Mae's rage elsewhere in the text, yet does not explore them: "Due to her improved capacity to deal with her husband, she understood how he provoked her rage and needed her to be raging and 'crazy'" (417). In addition to her husband, her father is mentioned: "She hoped for another pregnancy and for the first time, utilizing interpretation, began separating from her rage attacks. We saw these rage attacks as identification with her father, and she now remembered that her father repeatedly had attacks of rage to force his way with her or with her mother" (417).

Chessick does not, however, pursue the significance of these sources. This is evident in Chessick's analysis of an insight that Mae had during the sixth year of treatment: "The second half of the sixth year was marked by her slow recognition that she would not get physical holding from me, although she insisted that was all she wanted. At last she began therapeutic collaboration with discussion of her great rage as she approached men for 'love' and total mirroring admiration—smiling, warm approval of everything about her—and felt put down instead" (417).

Chessick's response to this is to offer what he terms a "deeper interpretation" of her rage. "A deeper interpretation of her rage is that it also defended her against the threat of the longed-for but much-feared symbiotic fusion with her mother. I did not interpret this directly out of my concern that even if she would be able to accept the interpretation, her shaky ego would become flooded by archaic longings and fears" (417).

Yet in the face of her turning to men for this fusion, Chessick reasons, "Her only hope of a warm relationship was with a man because there was nothing with her mother in the past. This dilemma was reinforced by her experience with her father, who combined physical warmth with physical abuse" (419).

But does Mae's insight speak more directly of her position in heterosexual gender relations, and the cultural ambivalence whereby women are both admired and devalued? The split that Chessick identifies in Mae's need for both fusion and revenge may be interpreted as a response to this ambivalent positioning of women. Mae's insight indicates her emerging awareness of her position. In response, Mae herself is split: "She claimed at this point that she was 'split down the middle'; one part wanted to give and be unfrigid and the other part kept a careful ledger and raged at all giving" (417).

This analysis reveals the main weakness of object relations theory:

its inability to account for the influence of the wider patriarchal culture, and specifically of the father as representative of that culture on the mother-infant dyad and on the child's construction of self as gendered. In this case, the exclusion of direct discussion of gender conflicts in Mae's construction of self leaves out important aspects of the world within which women are positioned.

This is evident in what is excluded from the case that would be pertinent to a more gendered reading: a direct discussion of her conflicts with men and her perception of her powerlessness and frustration in relation to them. Though there are repeated references to her husband, Chessick never takes up this issue directly, aiming his analysis instead on the pre-oedipal sources of Mae's rage and their manifestation in her present object relations as they are expressed in the therapy.

With the sole focus on the disastrous consequences of pre-oedipal deficits on Mae's psyche, specifically the lack of maternal warmth, no discussion appears regarding the lack of paternal warmth or intimacy and its effects on Mae's psyche. It is as if any warmth from her father, as a poor substitute for the mother, and even when mixed with abuse, is better than nothing. Yet in Chessick's framework, it is not expected and does not make up for the failures in her mother's care. This illustrates the cultural expectations that center on the mother while eliding the role of the father in direct relation to the child. But Chessick's theoretical orientation is not geared toward social relations, and thus his concern is to "firm up" Mae's sense of self, to be a "good enough mother" the way her own mother was not: "It was absolutely essential for me, in contrast to her mother, to give her emerging autonomous ego full latitude for growth, development, and regulation of her life" (417). By the seventh year of treatment progress is made as she begins developing an "observing ego" and a "control system that switched on even as rage flooded her" (417).

The workings of this displacement of paternal themes to maternal deprivation are not the workings of the conscious intentions of the analyst. The analyst's role in relation to the patient is fraught with ambivalence. He legitimates her narrative, and often adopts her point of view regarding her parents or her husband. Yet he participates in the power networks within which Mae constructs a self, by the assumptions that guide his interpretation of the root cause of her distress. In this case, it is the gap in the interpretation—the lack of acknowledgment of paternal power and control in this woman's life—that shapes his interpretation of her problems.

The analytic transfer or displacement of Mae's rage at men onto the pre-oedipal mother of object relations theory may serve a purpose for Chessick himself as an unconscious defense against this rage. Chessick's countertransferential reactions to it, evident in his statements about struggling not to get "sucked into the stormy chaos," or be "destroyed" by her raging, are resolved through this displacement of rage onto a destructive all-powerful mother.

This case differs from Ross's interpretation of Agnes's rage as completely without reason due to its embeddedness in an unconnected, fragmented narrative. Here the problem is not that the rage appears to be without reason—indeed, the reasons are abundant, as Mae offers a multitude of reasons for her rage. Yet Chessick, while acknowledging and reporting these reasons, seems always more concerned with what he sees as the real reason: the pre-oedipal mother as object representation, a reason gleaned from a "deeper interpretation," as he puts it. In Chessick's view, Mae's rage is not so much without reason as it is excessive, out of proportion to those reasons and therefore irrational. This case illustrates the construction of the borderline patient's rage as irrational and symptomatic of a character disorder.

Conclusion: Gender, Knowledge, and Perceptions of Anger in Women

> Anger is an emotion which must be reclaimed and legitimated as Woman's rightful, healthy expression—anger can be a source of power, strength and clarity as well as a creative force. (Juno and Vale 1991, 5)

This chapter analyzes the psychoanalytic interpretation of borderline patients' anger. In the psychoanalytical analysis this anger is portrayed as a flood of rage that overwhelms the analytic or therapeutic situation. These cases illustrate the psychoanalytic depiction of this rage as an inner disorganizing force and a sign of a breakdown of ego control. The women in these cases, Agnes and Mae, are portrayed as lacking stable selves, a condition attributed to their fundamental underlying mental pathology. Further, this underlying disease entity is said to be caused by the patient's prehistory rather than by her history.

This conflictual relationship may be understood as a struggle over knowledge. The cases illustrate this struggle; Agnes does not provide Ross with a coherent narrative, blocking his ability to know her; Ross, meanwhile, does not provide knowledge that is useful to Agnes. Similarly, Mae rejects Chessick's interpretation of her problems, while her flood of rage overwhelms their relationship and threatens Chessick's ability to maintain an analytic identity.

This chapter illustrates the way in which knowledge regarding the borderline patient is affected by the interactive context of the relationship between a borderline patient and her analyst. The intensity of the negative transference-countertransference dynamics of the borderline case—the anger and resistance manifested by the patient, and in turn, the responses of the analyst to this resistance—leads to the application of the borderline diagnosis, and the interpretation of the patient as lacking coherence. The borderline patient's refusal or resistance to the analytic situation puts that situation into crisis, decentering the analyst's position and interrupting the ritual work of interpretation. Borderline patients' anger appears to destabilize the analytic relationship and specifically to threaten the security of the analysts. Both Ross and Chessick express what Nathan Schwartz-Salant described as the sense of helplessness and the expectation of being attacked by the patient's anger, as well as the desire to flee from the patient. This instability and lack of coherence of the situation is then attributed to the patient, who is believed to harbor an underlying pathology that causes the patient's rage and that is at the root of the conflict between patient and analyst. Against this interpretation, the negative interaction characterizing these borderline cases is attributable, in a feminist interpretation, to the borderline patient's resistance to or refusal of the analytic situation and, more widely, to her position in patriarchal social relations. This feminist interpretation of the borderline patient is analogous to the feminist reinterpretation of hysteria, as illustrated by the differing analyses of Freud's case of Dora.

One specific epistemological effect of this conflictual analytic relation appearing in the text is the analytic displacement of borderline women's anger and resistance against male representatives of patriarchal power onto the pre-oedipal "bad mother." This analytic displacement or deflection of women's anger at male figures may represent the countertransferential defense of psychoanalysis against resistant or hostile patients, manifest here in the analyst's unconscious defense against the borderline patient's attacks against him.

In the battle of knowledge that these borderline cases represent, such attacks against the analyst's authority and knowledge are epistemological attacks as well. The patient's pre-oedipal mother is emphasized, while the patient's past and present oedipal relations (gender relations in the context of their contemporary arrangement) are elided.

The case texts, meanwhile, provide illustrative evidence of social, rather than pathological, sources of this anger. Such anger can be understood as women's response to their subordinate position in relations of knowledge and power. Borderline patients' anger may be understood as a response to the experience of therapy itself, a response based on their sensitivity to the scrutiny of therapy, and their overt rejection of analysts' interpretations of their particular problems.

The simultaneous social construction and neutralization (or pathologization) of this newly emerging anger in certain women patients is illustrative of the wider cultural construction of women who openly express anger as figures of disorder who are part of the realm of chaos, outside the boundaries of reasonable discourse. Rage is not considered to be part of the dominant conception of femininity. It is not perceived as one of the possible traits or reactions of a so-called normal woman. Normal women, in the Western cultural framework, are not supposed to feel anger, let alone express it. Indeed, many Western women express an inability to experience any anger. The cultural norms of femininity suggest that women more typically experience depression or self-directed feelings of hopelessness, shame, or guilt. Thus, rage and anger are, and have historically been, forbidden to women. Its expression is a sign, then, not only of a lack of femininity, but of a lack of mental stability. To the extent that women's normality as persons is bound up with their adherence to current norms of femininity, rage, as a flagrant transgression of these norms, puts the patient's mental stability as a person in doubt.

In this context, borderline women stand out as loud, demanding, repulsive, even monstrous—in their overt, active, vocal anger. Raging women appear both threatening and mad.

But when this symptom, rage, is read as politically meaningful, as an embodiment of contradictions in women's lives, it acquires a different meaning from that constructed in the psychomedical context. Rage is significant for women both as a transgression of dominant dictums of femininity and as a response to their social situation. The emergence of rage in increasing numbers of women who come to be diagnosed as borderline necessitates that we must identify the contradictory cultural conditions to which women's anger or rage is a response. Rage is becoming an increasingly central theme in women's lives and in diverse writings: rage rooted in women's feelings of powerlessness, rage at the persisting inequalities experienced by women, rage at the violence against women, at the need to feel fear; rage, also, as a potent anger that has been suppressed and has therefore acquired a certain force and intensity when it does finally emerge or erupt.

This may be why, for many women, rage is experienced as empowerment—it is as though an injustice has been named and some primal truth reached; some boundary has been crossed and the acquiescence or subordination has been cast aside. bell hooks quotes a line from Toni Morrison's *The Bluest Eye*: "Anger is better—there is a presence in anger." Commenting, hooks says, "I was always moved by that contrasting of victimization vs. being victimized; it's important to maintain the kind of rage that allows you to resist" (hooks 1991, 81).

Many borderline patients state that feeling anger or rage makes them feel alive and helps them break through a feeling of being dead inside. "I am finally able to be a 5, previously I was either a 0 or a 10. I had to have very strong feelings in order to feel alive. I had to feel very deeply about other people, to have very intense contempt or rage, or feel this about myself. Then I was alive. Now I am beginning to have more normal feelings, to hate my husband but also feel some care as well. Previously this was impossible. I had to start fights to feel alive. Anything that approached a 5 was too frightening. It meant I would feel dead" (Schwartz-Salant 1987, 52).

Thus rage is culturally significant for women at this historical juncture. To map out its historical significance, it is necessary to reframe such "pathological" rage as a response, and an initial resistance, against social injustice—against, in other words, social denigration, devaluation, or distortion.

The object relations psychoanalytic approach takes an initial step toward a social interpretation of psychic conflicts. This approach is manifest in the strategy of treating the patient's relationship to therapy and to the therapist as a microcosm of the patient's overall relationship to others. In these cases, the opportunity exists for analysts to pursue this approach far enough to connect their patients' anger to their gender position. However, in the cases presented here, gender relations are not pursued as significant sources of women's anger, and analysts focus their interpretation on the patient's inner, pre-oedipal dynamics. The effect of this oversight is to reproduce the construction of women's anger as pathological and irrational, rather than as an intelligible response to their social situation.

Chapter 6	Conclusion

Gender and the
Politics of Madness

I T HAS BEEN the goal of this book to analyze the narrative construction of the meaning of the borderline category within psychoanalytic psychiatry, and to trace the history of its feminization in the clinical discourse. This analysis demonstrates that the relationship between gender and the borderline category is socially constructed from several currents. As the historical review of the evolution of the term shows, the borderline construct is an assemblage of disparate symptoms and psychodynamic formulations, brought together in an artificial unity. This is thus an illustration of psychiatry's role in constructing its own object of inquiry (Kovel 1988).

The grouping of diverse symptoms into the unity known as borderline personality disorder is partially a construction of psychiatric discourse itself, a discourse that makes sense of women's conflicts through the lens of the ambiguous and elusive concept of the borderland between sanity and madness. Yet the therapeutic applications of the borderline label to specific women do not totally determine the phenomenon. To view the borderline diagnosis as a mere label neglects the depth of the suffering of women seeking treatment for their psychic distress. The borderline is, rather, the effect of the intersection between women's socially produced responses to the construction of gender, and the psychiatric discourse of the "psy complex" (Ingleby 1985).

The immediate social context for this intersection of women and

psychiatric discourse is the therapeutic situation, a contradictory relationship marked by both the hegemony of scientific rationality and the
benevolence and paternalism of the psy complex. This mix of control
and care, in which the management of women's individual disorder is
at the same time reflective of women's dependence on therapeutic
frameworks, structures the meaning made of the borderline malady. As
the case narratives have shown, the therapeutic relationship is also one
marked by intense transferential currents of tension, unease, and rage,
and this transferential dimension interrupts and destabilizes the interpretive work of psychiatric rituals.

The borderline concept refers not only to the borders between madness and sanity, but to the cultural borders that psychiatry is called on
to legislate in order to define that crucial border of sanity. The cases
demonstrate the way in which women's transgressions across borders
(between the therapeutic and the personal; between self and other; between the human and the inhuman or uncanny; between sexual normality and promiscuity; between normal emotion and inappropriate
rage) are interpreted as signs of mental pathology. In the conflicted setting of the therapeutic relationship, the definition of the boundaries of
madness and sanity is also the legislation of appropriate selfhood for
women. The narratives, then, are scenes of the negotiation of meaning
of women's subjectivity in a relationship of power and resistance.

Within the discourse on the borderline personality, the concept of
the unified and coherent self is the standard against which the borderline patient is measured. The borderline patient's self is perceived as
insufficiently distinguished from its surroundings, intangible, or fragmented; this fragmentation is postulated as an inner pathology caused
by deficient mothering. The metaphors of liquidity and fluidity that
analysts use to describe the unstable or raging self draws upon and reproduces the cultural disquiet about the leakiness and formlessness of
femininity. The rhetorical construction of the borderline, then, is similar
to the way hysteria was described in the nineteenth century: as unruly,
emotionally labile and capricious, a "perverse or hyper femininity," in
the words of Carroll Smith-Rosenberg (1972).

An examination of the types of people to whom the appellation
"borderline" has been applied over the course of its history shows that

it is a symbol for the marginal, the uncategorizable—frequently, the deviant or resistant patient who cannot otherwise be categorized or diagnosed. This trope of the marginal and fragmentary comes to be applied to certain women (and some men) in the bounds of the therapeutic setting.

Another common element linking the heterogeneous group that is designated borderline is that these patients resist smooth uninterrupted psychoanalytic interpretation or psychotherapeutic alliance. They are unanalyzable—silent, providing no flow of talk, no free association; uncanny, strange, mechanical or inhuman. Or they resist more overtly, blocking each interpretive gesture made by their analysts, maintaining their rage, thereby maintaining a rejection of the analytic/therapeutic complex within which they come to be defined as borderline.

As applied to specific women, the term becomes a signifier for the female patient with symptoms that are difficult to manage or analyze, symptoms that may be more intelligible as responses to women's contemporary social situation. In addition, these symptoms are diverse, ranging from emptiness, numbness, and passivity, to uncertainty of self-image, to so-called promiscuity and rage. As the cases have shown, the borderline diagnosis is applied to very different types of women. In addition, heterogeneous symptoms within the same woman come to be perceived as signs of an underlying instability—a stably unstable disorder. In this sense, the borderline label appears to indeed be a contemporary successor to hysteria as a heterogeneous category of pathology in women.

The case narratives portray these resistances as signs of an inner pathological instability, a sign of an intangible, fluid, or incoherent self. Yet the discussion of cases of men who receive the borderline diagnosis reveals that they are interpreted not as unstable, but as rigid, defensive, and hypervigilant, a stance that resembles culturally defined standards of masculinity. However, those men who display lapses in this hegemonic masculinity are also portrayed as unstable. The narratives of male patients illustrate that gender discourse is operative in the ways men are deemed pathological also, and confirm Joan Busfield's contention that men may be labeled for exaggerated or nonconforming expressions of masculinity (Busfield 1996).

Women's Madness as Resistance

One of the most important aspects of a feminist critique and decon-struction of the meanings of women's madness is its critical challenge to social norms of femininity, normality, and mental health that un-derlie the "regime of self" in late modern society. This study has sug-gested that norms of selfhood, embedded in the formal psychoanalytic theoretical narratives, are renegotiated in the narratives of borderline patients. Faced with patients who appear to lack recognizable selves, analysts narrativize these more complex and fragmented subjectivities in their case descriptions. Borderline patients' symptoms can be read as signs of cultural and social ills, through an analysis that depathologizes and politicizes them, placing them in the larger context of gender and power. It is important to read symptoms as signs not only of individual women's suffering or dis-ease, but also of the culture—its contradictions, tensions, and oppressions. It is akin to Susan Bordo's approach to ana-lyzing anorexia as the "crystallization of culture." She writes, "I take the psychopathologies that develop within a culture, far from being anoma-lies or aberrations, to be characteristic expressions of that culture; to be, indeed, the crystallization of much that is wrong with it. For that reason they are important to examine, as keys to cultural self-diagnosis and self-scrutiny" (Bordo 1993, 141).

In their analyses of women's madness as a form of resistance, Bordo (1993), Cixous and Clément (1986), and Ong (1988) show the com-plex negotiation of experience that women's madness represents, that, while appearing to collude with the disciplinary networks of power within which they find themselves, also represents a form of uncon-scious resistance. In a recent analysis of feminist literary interpretations of madness in women, Marta Caminero-Santangelo criticizes the strat-egy of reading women's madness as protest (Caminero-Santangelo 1998). She objects to feminist literary interpretations of women's texts that valorize and even champion women's madness as a potentially liberatory means of protest. Contrary to what these valorizations of women's madness suggest, she argues, madness is a sign not of protest or resistance, but of women's ultimate powerlessness, signaling the mo-ment of capitulation to power. In the feminist analyses, madness "pro-vides the illusion of power while locating the mad (non)subject outside any sphere where power can be located" (4). She argues that more attention must be paid to how women themselves understand their condition and reject it as disempowering. Women who write autobiographically about their own madness, she suggests, are not doing so in order to celebrate madness as a means of resistance; rather, they are writing about the ultimate powerlessness of madness and about their discovery of other means of escape or resolution to their conflicts.

It is also important to stress that a strategic feminist reading of women's madness as intelligible or meaningful in a context of gender relations is not the same as a suggestion that such responses are laudable or preferable to other responses. Indeed, many feminist critics seem to be at pains to point out the futility of madness as a response. Susan Bordo, for example, argues against a simplistic celebration of the liberatory aspects of madness: "Although we may talk meaningfully of protest, then, I want to emphasize the counterproductive, tragically self-defeating (indeed, self-deconstructing) nature of that protest. Functionally, the symptoms of these disorders isolate, weaken, and undermine the sufferers; at the same time they turn the life of the body into an all-absorbing fetish, beside which all other objects of attention pale into unreality. On the symbolic level, too, the protest collapses into its opposite and proclaims the utter capitulation of the subject to the contracted female world" (Bordo 1993, 176). What feminist analyses do offer, then, is a way to understand women's madness as an intelligible response to unlivable conditions in which other modes of response are blocked off.

What Caminero-Santangelo makes more audible in feminist analyses is the importance of remembering women's psychic pain, a pain that women experiencing it seek help in ending. Feminist critics, then, must make more explicit the implications of their critiques for women's psychic lives, individually and collectively. As Jane Ussher writes, it is crucial to advance critical analysis beyond critique: "The critiques of the antipsychiatrists and feminists have their place. They challenge directly our taken-for-granted assumptions about the world, about women, and about madness. But this is not enough, for they negate the importance of the individual woman trapped within the system which pronounces upon her condition in paternalistic and patronizing ways. They deny women who need an answer, who have no voice; women who find little comfort in the deconstructions and find that the tranquilizers dull the pain" (Ussher 1992, 291).

Reimagining the Borders: Implications of Deconstructing the Borderline Diagnosis

What are the implications of this analysis for clinical practices themselves, for those who practice the arts of helping, including making diagnostic judgments and plans for treating women who seek help? What might a feminist critical analysis of the meaning of the borderline category suggest for those whose work is dedicated to helping women, and for women themselves, who seek help in relieving or understanding their pain?

First, there are direct implications for clinical practice of deconstructing the category itself. A major task suggested by this analysis for those who practice the art of helping is to first question the self-evidence or transparent reality of the category of borderline disorder as an entity, as represented in the DSM-IV. The complex and changing history of the category shows that it is highly questionable to understand its contemporary manifestation as a singular entity that someone could be said to simply "have." And as Dana Becker points out, determining whether a patient has or does not have borderline personality disorder is not very helpful in guiding treatment, since it is such a heterogeneous category that it does not refer to a singular entity (Becker 1997, 159). She suggests a more nuanced, dimensional model of assessing an individual's symptoms, as has been suggested by Trull, Widiger, and Guthrie (1990). Their analysis of 409 psychiatric hospital charts suggested that borderline syndrome should be conceptualized "as a dimensional variable with persons varying in the extent to which they display borderline psychopathology, rather than to categorize persons arbitrarily as borderline or not borderline" (46). Becker notes that such an approach can be more individually attuned to the specific needs of patients, "without recourse to the use of labels" (Becker 1997, 159).

Joel Kovel offers another perspective from which to consider the role of diagnostic categories in light of the contemporary dominance of the DSM in mental health practice. The DSM, Kovel argues, reifies the disease model of mental illness as a bounded, inner diathesis. Its use can have a dehumanizing effect on the patient, when the practitioner places emphasis on the disorder as an abstract thing. The patient is thus viewed in a decontextualized fashion, outside the social and historical contexts within which her or his symptoms have meaning. For change to occur, the focus must be upon "the person and his/her relation to the world—instead of being located in the false abstraction of mental disorder" (Kovel 1988, 145).

Kovel makes it clear that he is not against diagnosis as a useful part of psychotherapy. Diagnosis can help to organize knowledge about a patient, enabling the clinician to understand previously unrelated elements. The problem comes, however, when diagnosis is divorced from the social relationship between a therapist and patient, and becomes an abstraction. "For there is no such thing as diagnosis in the abstract. There is only concrete diagnosing as a social practice" (131). Given this, Kovel argues that the therapist should see her/himself as the primary "instrument" for creating meaning about a patient's condition, rather than for establishing a diagnostic classification. "We are insisting then that the psychiatrist himself is the instrument, and that he is not outside of what he does and learns" (145). Clinicians must maintain a reflexive awareness of how they are making use of the borderline category, for which types of patients and for which specific interactions.

Clinicians must also be aware of the kind of language that is used and circulated in describing those patients deemed borderline. As this analysis has shown, and as many critics within the clinical literature have pointed out, much of this language is inherently pejorative. "Such terms as manipulative, seductive, controlling, needy, devouring, frigid, castrating, masochistic, and hysterical have been used pervasively, primarily to describe female patients" (Becker 1997, 150). Marcia Linehan writes of the effect of this pejorative language on treatment:

> It seems to me that such pejorative terms do not themselves increase compassion, understanding, and a caring attitude for borderline patients. Instead, for many therapists such terms create emotional distance from and anger at borderline individuals. . . . One of the main goals of my theoretical endeavors has been to develop a theory of BPD that is both scientifically sound and nonjudgemental and nonpejorative in tone.

The idea here is that such a theory should lead to effective treatment techniques as well as to a compassionate attitude. Such an attitude is needed, especially with this population: Our tools to help them are limited; their misery is intense and vocal; and the success or failure of our attempts to help can have extreme outcomes. (Linehan 1993, 18)

This questioning of the borderline category entails a shift in how past case histories of borderline disorder are read. Rather than being understood as veritable accounts of the analysis of an actually existing disorder, they must be read provisionally, as constructed narratives, created in the contexts of both existing psychological and psychiatric theory and the gendered interactions of therapist and patient. Thus, therapists should have a familiarity with the history of the borderline concept in order to recognize its shifting, constructed character. This would help them to avoid the tendency to view the borderline as an unchanging single entity. Their familiarity with its pejorative connotations could help them see that when they use it, they should do so carefully and with an awareness of its potential linkages to negative views of their patients.

The recent tendency to use popular films as models of borderline personality disorder in the teaching of medical students can only further increase the confusion regarding how the category of borderline is understood (Hyler and Schanzer 1997; Wedding and Boyd 1999). Many of the film characters used as examples of women with borderline personality disorder are reductive stereotypes, created within film narratives that are, as in the case of *Fatal Attraction*, highly misogynist and reactionary in the political and social contexts within which they have been created. These powerful visual images can only magnify the pejorative overtones of the borderline diagnosis when it is applied to women.

Another crucial implication for responding to symptoms that come to be called borderline is for clinicians, patients, and observers at large to understand that those symptoms are intimately connected to the contradictions and violence of gender in late modern culture. We must understand that those women seeking help who are experiencing numbness, dissociation, or subjective confusion; or who are expressing extreme anger or psychic pain; or who are self-mutilating or suicidal, are responding to the erasures, denials, repression and suppression of self, powerlessness, and often victimization of violence or sexual abuse, in a world of gender and power. This shift in understanding can significantly affect the ways these so-called symptoms are understood and treated.

The feminist treatment models of clinicians such as Judith Herman, Dana Becker, Marcia Linehan, and Jane Flax, are all oriented toward the crucial importance of situating women's symptoms in this larger context of gender. Further, each of them questions the value placed on the norm of a bounded, autonomous self as a marker of mental health, showing how this privileges a culturally defined masculine mode of being and devalues dependence upon others as inherently unhealthy.

For Judith Herman, the experience of physical violence or sexual abuse is an important factor to which clinicians must pay attention in their overall assessment of the patient. Herman's work on post-traumatic stress disorder provides a framework for understanding a patient's behaviors as responses to past abuse, rather than as manifestations of the patient's "presumed underlying psychopathology" (Herman 1992, 116). This can have the effect of rehumanizing the potentially dehumanizing and pejorative connotations of the borderline diagnosis.

However, as Dana Becker notes, early childhood events of abuse cannot be viewed as the sole determining factor in the heterogeneous group of patients who receive the borderline diagnosis. Becker argues for a more broadly construed gender context in understanding the symptoms deemed borderline. "What would contribute substantially toward improved treatment of women called 'borderline' would be the increasing ability of clinicians to understand the relationship between 'borderline' symptoms and female socialization" (Becker 1997, 159). Becker focuses on girls' construction of self in adolescence, in particular, arguing that the social environment for girls negatively affects their self-esteem and overall mental well-being. "Overall, it would appear, coming of age in our culture poses more risks for adolescent girls than for adolescent boys" (96). One of the central aspects of this female socialization is the emphasis placed on relatedness, nurturance, and other-directedness in girls, ways of being that are devalued in the culture at large. Because of the high value placed upon autonomy and separateness as signs of a healthy self, women are being socialized into a self that is viewed as unhealthy and overdependent on others. Further, since they are encouraged to rely on others for validation of the self, they develop a "magnified self-consciousness and consequent increase in fear of displeasing others. This results in a greater sensitivity to criticism or disapproval, generally, than exists in boys. . . . Uncertainty in women may have its origins in the dependence on others for validation of self-worth" (96).

Psychotherapist Harriet Lerner argues that one crucial element of therapy with women is the assumption that the patient's sensitivity or concern regarding the gendered social and cultural roots of her difficulties is a legitimate and important focus of treatment. Lerner notes that while most therapists do indeed focus on both intrapsychic and sociocultural dimensions of their patients' problems, they differ in the stress placed on these aspects.

> There still exists much controversy about whether women who angrily protest societal definitions of femininity and the feminine role are themselves expressing neurotic conflicts, or whether, on the other hand, it is our very definitions of femininity and the feminine role that are the pathogenesis of female symptomatology. This is not simply a matter of theoretical interest, for a therapist's position regarding this controversy (whether conscious and explicit or unexamined and unconsciously held) determines the very course and process of treatment, despite that therapist's very best intentions to "help patients make their own choices" in an atmosphere that is "value free." (Lerner 1988, 124)

If clinicians understood the influence of female socialization in shaping their clients' behaviors, argues Becker, they would be less inclined to perceive them as "manipulative" or "hostile," terms that are inherently pejorative and that have been commonly used to describe female patients (Becker 1997).

If symptoms deemed borderline are understood as responses to gender socialization, what does this imply for developing strategies for helping women who experience them? One treatment approach that has been hailed as successful is aimed directly at women's self-destructive thoughts and behaviors, teaching them skills to intervene in negative feelings and to replace them with alternatives. This is Dialectical Behavioral Therapy, developed by Marcia Linehan (1993). It is based on Linehan's belief that the most salient target for change in women with symptoms deemed borderline is to enhance their own awareness of and responses to their negative, self-destructive emotions. Persons who express the behaviors that are grouped under the borderline label may have had invalidating, and sometimes abusive, childhood family and social environments, which disrupt their creation of a positive sense of identity. Because borderline symptoms are more frequent in women, Linehan cites a sexist society as a major source of invalidation. However, Linehan notes, not all women become borderline. "Certainly, sexism is an important source of invalidation for all women in our culture; just as certainly, all women do not become borderline. Nor do all women with vulnerable temperaments become borderline, even though all women are exposed to sexism in one form or another" (52). Linehan cites other factors that may be present, including sexual abuse; a failure by parents to imitate their infant's emotional expressions; the cultural devaluation of a child's dependence upon others as "unhealthy"; and overt sexism in which female children are punished for displaying "unfeminine" behaviors or skills (55). Linehan also incorporates biological factors into her model, arguing that a foundation for developing borderline symptoms is a predisposition to sensitivity and emotional vulnerability. However, the treatment is not aimed at biology, but at cognition and behaviors that patients can learn in order to develop new, less self-destructive responses to their psychological pain. As one psychologist who has developed an outpatient treatment program for adolescent borderline patients notes, "Other people have learned how to take care of themselves emotionally, how to self-soothe. Borderlines have not. . . . It is what other people do all the time, for borderlines—who never learned the basics of emotional and verbal negotiation, these things have to be explicitly taught" (Kornreich 1997, 16).

While the dialectical model shares many features of cognitive behavioral therapy, it also uses a framework of "dialectics" that Linehan defines as "the reconciliation of opposites in a continual process of synthesis. . . . The most fundamental dialectic is the necessity of accepting patients just as they are within a context of trying to teach them to change" (Linehan 1993, 19). Linehan notes that she draws from Zen Buddhism to emphasize both the necessity of change and the acceptance of what is. Hence, dialectical behavioral treatment is distinguished by its greater level of support to the patient (they are permitted to make phone calls to the therapist between sessions). In addition, therapists work in teams so that they can help support each other (Kornreich 1997, 16).

Significantly, the dialectical approach forgoes a focus on the separate, independent and bounded self in favor of a more contextual view of the person, one resembling in Linehan's description a poststructural understanding of identity: "Identity itself is relational, and boundaries between parts are temporary and exist only in relation to the whole; indeed, it is the whole that determines the boundaries" (Linehan 1993, 31).

Linehan points out that the cultural value placed on independent and bounded selfhood informs conceptions of mental health, so that normality is equated with independence, while interdependence is devalued and pathologized as unhealthy. Given that women are socialized to be more dependent and to define themselves in relation to others, their modes of being in the world are not valued in the culture at large, nor within dominant modes of mental health. Thus "the problems encountered by the borderline individual may result in part from the collision of a relational self with a society that recognizes and rewards only the individuated self" (32).

Linehan's contextual, dialectical approach also forgoes a certainty about fixed "truth." The focus on ongoing change means that "truth" is never absolute; it "evolves, develops, and is constructed over time. From the dialectical perspective, nothing is self-evident, and nothing stands apart from anything else as unrelated knowledge. The spirit of a dialectical point of view is never to accept a final truth or an undisputable fact. Thus, the question addressed by both patient and therapist is 'What is being left out of our understanding?'" (35).

Jane Flax offers a feminist interpretation of her patient Laurie's fragmentation by looking to the cultural repression of women's autonomy and sexual agency as sources of Laurie's psychic divisions and splitting. In a recent discussion, Flax goes further in drawing out the implications of a feminist, poststructural understanding of subjectivity for psychoanalytic practice. Flax argues that it is necessary to make a radical shift away from a language of self and toward one of multiple and shifting subjectivities. "Language to discuss multiple subjectivity requires terms with less bounded or solid connotations than 'self.' Subjectivity is a complex verb rather than a noun" (Flax 1996, 578). Just as Flax discourages the adherence to fixed theoretical "lines" or narratives of the self, she emphasizes openness and more dynamic criteria for "success" in therapy outcomes. "*Be prepared to be surprised* might be the motto of a postmodernist analyst" (588). Rather than being encouraged to find fixed meaning in their lives, patients are encouraged to accept its radical contingency, its elusive quality. In a passage that resonates with Linehan's conception of Zen acceptance, Flax writes, "The patient learns that he or she can live with multiple, often contradictory stories and develops the capacity to revise them as necessary in ongoing life struggles. At least as important, the patient learns to tolerate the absence of meaning, the limits of narrative organization, and the ineradicable persistence of unintelligibility. The capacity to construct meaning or story lines, like all human powers, is finite. Some events or experiences happen randomly or are too horrible to comprehend. Sometimes we confront experiences that simply are; we cannot make sense of them, fit them into a believable story line, or understand their causes. . . . We can only register their existence and some of their effects on us" (589).

Flax's position may be viewed as part of a growing interest in and development of what are variously called narrative, social constructionist, or postmodern forms of psychotherapy. Within psychoanalysis proper, analysts such as Irwin Hoffman argue that a new paradigm is emerging, one that goes beyond the shift toward a relational conception of psychoanalysis described by Greenberg and Mitchell (1983). This new paradigm is predicated on a critique of the positivist, realist assumptions that underlie analytic practice, and views whatever truths that emerge to be constructed interactively by both analyst and patient (Hoffman 1991).

In psychology too, narrative therapies, drawing upon social constructionist and postmodern theoretical frameworks in the social sciences for therapy, have been developed (Freedman and Combs 1996; McNamee and Gergen 1992; White and Epston 1990). What is needed, as Gergen and Kaye argue, is a view of therapy as a "process of *semiosis*:

the forging of meaning in the context of collaborative discourse" (Gergen and Kaye 1992, 182). If therapy consists of the joint construction of meaning, then the role of the therapist necessarily must shift. Rather than viewing one's role as expert knower, the therapist becomes a cocreator of meaning, engaged in a "receptive mode of inquiry" characterized by "openness to different ways of punctuating experience, readiness to explore multiple perspectives and endorse their coexistence" (182–83).

The narrative or constructionist approach implies changes in how past childhood sexual or physical abuse is regarded in the present. While the narrative therapist takes this past experience seriously, s/he does not view it as an invariant truth that the client must reexperience in order to be helped. Truth is not viewed as something to be discovered; rather, attention is paid to the joint construction of its meaning. Under this approach, attention shifts away from asking the client to reexperience the past. As William Hudson O'Hanlon writes, "Current approaches to the treatment of the after-effects of sexual abuse hold that they are discovering and uncovering the truth about client's childhoods. They also imply that the only way to help clients resolve these issues is to remember, tell, and express the feelings and incidents they repressed involving the abuse" (O'Hanlon 1992, 137). In contrast, O'Hanlon notes, clients and therapists cocreate the problem to be worked upon, and the therapists influence the ways in which patients remember and relate these experiences. Therapy should orient not toward a recall of actual events, but toward the creation of new ways of viewing these memories, as they are currently narrated.

In the narrative or postmodern approaches, the patient's perspective on the world is taken seriously, on its own terms, and the position of the therapist is reoriented so the therapist is able to give greater attention to the patient's voice, as in Linehan's dialectical acceptance. Further, like Flax, Gergen and Kaye wish to press beyond the creation of new narratives for the patient, and argue for fostering a new awareness of the multiplicity and contingency of all narratives. As they write, "It is a progression from learning new meanings, to developing new categories of meaning, to transforming one's premises about the nature of meaning itself" (Gergen and Kaye 1992, 182). When one gives up on singular, fixed conceptions of selfhood as markers of psychological health, then the underlying, ongoing process of subjectivity emerges. For Gergen and Kaye, it is a continual embrace of relatedness: "If there is identity at this level, it cannot be articulated, laid out for public view in a given description or explanation. It lies in the boundless and inarticulable capacity for relatedness itself" (181).

It may be objected that such prescriptions for treatment of the symptoms labeled borderline amounts to an acceptance of the existence of an inner diathesis, which this book has explicitly argued against. However, we need not simply accept a disease model for so-called border- lines. Rather, we may view their self-destructive feelings and behaviors as lying at the extreme end of a range of responses to gender contra- dictions and violence in late modern society. This does not mean that all women are potentially borderline. However, it does call attention to the continuum of feminine dis-ease in the culture, and to its sources in the social organization of gender. While we are developing a means to help women at its extreme end cope with their lives and feelings, we must also attend to the need for changes in that organization of gen- der, to an explicitly feminist revaluation and refiguration of what it means to be woman in late modern society.

References

Abend, Sander M., Michael S. Porder, and Martin S. Willick. 1983. *Borderline Patients: Psychoanalytic Perspectives*. New York: International Universities Press.

American Psychiatric Association. 1980. *Diagnostic and Statistical Manual of Mental Disorders, Third Edition*. Washington, D.C.: American Psychiatric Association.

———.1987. *Diagnostic and Statistical Manual of Mental Disorders, Third Edition—Revised*. Washington, D.C.: American Psychiatric Association.

———.1994. *Diagnostic and Statistical Manual of Mental Disorders, Fourth Edition*. Washington, D.C.: American Psychiatric Association.

Aronson, Thomas A. 1985. "Historical Perspectives on the Borderline Concept: A Review and Critique." *Psychiatry* 48: 209–222.

Astbury, Jill. 1996. *Crazy for You: The Making of Women's Madness*. Oxford, U.K.: Oxford University Press.

Babener, Liahna. 1992. "Patriarchal Politics in *Fatal Attraction*." *Journal of Popular Culture* 26: 25–34.

Beauvoir, Simone de. 1989. *The Second Sex*. Trans. E. M. Parshley. New York: Vintage.

Becker, Dana. 1997. *Through the Looking Glass: Women and Borderline Personality Disorder*. Boulder, Colo.: Westview Press.

Benjamin, Jessica. 1988. *The Bonds of Love: Psychoanalysis, Feminism, and the Problem of Domination*. New York: Pantheon Books.

Bernheimer, Charles, and Claire Kahane. 1985. *In Dora's Case: Freud-Hysteria-Feminism*. New York: Columbia University Press.

Blashfield, Roger K., and Ross A. McElroy. 1987. "The 1985 Journal Literature on the Personality Disorders." *Comprehensive Psychiatry* 28 (6): 536–546.

Bordo, Susan. 1986. "The Cartesian Masculinization of Thought." *Signs* 11 (3): 439–456.

———.1993. *Unbearable Weight: Feminism, Western Culture, and the Body*. Berkeley: University of California Press.

Boyer, Bryce L. 1977. "Working with a Borderline Patient." *Psychoanalytic Quarterly* 46: 386–424.

Brooks, Peter. 1984. *Reading for the Plot*. New York: Alfred A. Knopf.

Brown, Philip. 1990. "The Name Game: Toward a Sociology of Diagnosis." *Journal of Mind and Behavior* 11 (3–4): 385–406.

Bruner, Jerome. 1987. "Life as Narrative." *Social Research* 54 (1): 11–32.

Busfield, Joan. 1996. *Men, Women and Madness: Understanding Gender and Mental Disorder*. New York: New York University Press.

Butler, Judith. 1990. *Gender Trouble: Feminism and the Subversion of Identity*. New York: Routledge.

———.1993. *Bodies That Matter: On the Discursive Limits of Sex*. New York: Routledge.

Caminero-Santangelo, Marta. 1998. *The Madwoman Can't Speak: Or Why Insanity Is Not Subversive*. Ithaca: Cornell University Press.

Castaneda, Ricardo, and Hugo Franco. 1985. "Sex and Ethnic Distribution of Borderline Personality Disorder in an Inpatient Sample." *American Journal of Psychiatry* 142 (2): 1202–1203.

Cauwels, Janice. 1992. *Imbroglio: Rising to the Challenges of Borderline Personality Disorder*. New York: W. W. Norton.

Cheever, Susan. 1993. "A Designated Crazy." *New York Times Book Review*, 20 June, 1, 24.

Chesler, Phyllis. 1989. *Women and Madness*. Orlando: Harcourt Brace Jovanovich.

Chessick, Richard. 1966. "The Psychotherapy of Borderland Patients." *American Journal of Psychotherapy* 20: 600–614.

———.1972. "Externalization and Existential Anguish in the Borderline Patient." *Archives of General Psychiatry* 27 (6): 764–771.

———.1977. *Intensive Psychotherapy of the Borderline Patient*. New York: Jason Aronson.

———.1982. "Intensive Psychotherapy of a Borderline Patient." *Archives of General Psychiatry* 39: 413–419.

Cixous, Hélène, and Catherine Clément. 1986. *The Newly Born Woman*. Trans. B. Wing. Minneapolis: University of Minnesota Press.

Clément, Catherine. 1986. "The Guilty One." In *The Newly Born Woman*, by H. Cixous and C. Clément. Trans. B. Wing. Minneapolis: University of Minnesota Press.

———.1987. *The Weary Sons of Freud*. New York: Verso.

Clifford, James. 1986. "Introduction: Partial Truths." In *Writing Culture: The Poetics and Politics of Ethnography*. Eds. J. Clifford and G. E. Marcus. Berkeley: University of California Press.

Cohn, Carol. 1995. "Wars, Wimps and Women: Talking Gender and Thinking War." In *Men's Lives*. Ed. M. S. Kimmel and M. A. Messner. Boston: Allyn and Bacon.

Davis, Kathe. 1992. "The Allure of the Predatory Woman in *Fatal Attraction* and Other Current American Movies." *Journal of Popular Culture* 26: 47–57.

De Chenne, Timothy. 1991. "Diagnosis as Therapy for the Borderline Personality." *Psychotherapy* 28 (2): 284–291.

de Lauretis, Teresa. 1984. *Alice Doesn't: Feminism, Semiotics, Cinema*. Bloomington: Indiana University Press.

Denzin, Norman. 1997. *Interpretive Ethnography: Ethnographic Practices for the 21st Century*. Thousand Oaks, Calif.: Sage.

Deutsch, Helene. 1942. "Some Forms of Emotional Disturbance and Their Relationship to Schizophrenia." In *Essential Papers on Borderline Disorders: One Hundred Years at the Border*. Ed. M. H. Stone. New York: New York University Press.

Fairclough, Norman. 1989. *Language and Power*. London: Longman.

Fee, Dwight. 1999. "The Broken Dialogue: Mental Illness as Discourse and Experience." In *Pathology and the Postmodern: Mental Illness as Discourse and Experience*. Ed. D. Fee. London: Sage.

Ferguson, Kathy. 1991. "Interpretation and Genealogy in Feminism." *Signs* 16: 322–339.

Flax, Jane. 1986. "Re-Membering the Selves: Is the Repressed Gendered?" *Michigan Quarterly Review* 26: 92–110.

———.1996. "Taking Multiplicity Seriously: Some Implications for Psychoanalytic Theorizing and Practice." *Contemporary Psychoanalysis* 32 (4): 577–593.

Foucault, Michel. 1965. *Madness and Civilization: A History of Insanity in the Age of Reason*. New York: Vintage Books.

———.1980. *History of Sexuality: Volume I: An Introduction*. Trans. R. Hurley. New York: Vintage.

———.1984. "Nietzsche, Genealogy, History." In *The Foucault Reader*. Ed. P. Rabinow. New York: Pantheon Books.

Freedman, Jill, and Gene Combs. 1996. *Narrative Therapy : The Social Construction of Preferred Realities*. New York: W. W. Norton.

Freud, Sigmund. 1963 (1905). *Dora: An Analysis of a Case of Hysteria*. Ed. P. Reiff. New York: Collier.

Frosh, Stephen. 1987. *The Politics of Psychoanalysis: An introduction to Freudian and Post-Freudian Theory*. New Haven, Conn.: Yale University Press.

———.1991. *Identity Crisis: Modernity, Psychoanalysis and the Self*. New York: Routledge.

Gallop, Jane. 1982. *The Daughter's Seduction: Feminism and Psychoanalysis*. Ithaca, N.Y.: Cornell University Press.

———.1985. *Reading Lacan*. Ithaca, N.Y.: Cornell University Press.

Gallop, Ruth, W. J. Lancee, and Paul Garfinkel. 1989. "How Nursing Staff Respond to the Label 'Borderline Personality Disorder.'" *Hospital and Community Psychiatry* 40 (8): 815–819.

Gelfond, Marjorie. 1991. "Reconceptualizing Agoraphobia: A Case Study of Epistemological Bias in Clinical Research." *Feminism and Psychology* 1 (2): 247–262.

Gergen, Kenneth. 1991. *The Saturated Self: Dilemmas of Identity in Contemporary Life*. New York: Basic Books.

Gergen, Kenneth J., and John Kaye. 1992. "Beyond Narrative in Negotiation of Meaning." In *Therapy As Social Construction*. Ed. S. McNamee and K. J. Gergen. Thousand Oaks, Calif.: Sage.

Gibson, Diane. 1991. "Borderline Personality Disorder: Issues of Etiology and Gender." *Occupational Therapy in Mental Health* 10 (4): 63–77.

Green, André. 1977. "The Borderline Concept: A Conceptual Framework for the Understanding of Borderline Patients: Suggested Hypotheses." In *Borderline Disorders: the Concept, the Syndrome, the Patient*. Ed. P. Hartcollis. New York: International Universities Press.

Greenberg, J. R., and S. A. Mitchell. 1983. *Object Relations in Psychoanalytic Theory*. Cambridge, Mass.: Harvard University Press.

Griggers, Camilla. 1997. *Becoming Woman*. Minneapolis: University of Minnesota Press.

Grosz, Elizabeth. 1994. *Volatile Bodies: Toward a Corporeal Feminism*. Bloomington: Indiana University Press.

Gunderson, John G., and Mary C. Zanarini. 1987. "Current Overview of the Borderline Diagnosis." *Journal of Clinical Psychiatry* 48: 5–11.

Henry, K. A., and C. I. Cohen. 1983. "The Role of Labeling Processes in Diagnosing Borderline Personality Disorder." *American Journal of Psychiatry* 140 (11): 1527–1529.

Herman, Andrew. 1999. *The Better Angels of Capitalism: Rhetoric, Narrative and Moral Identity Among Men of the Upper Class*. Boulder, Colo.: Westview Press.

Herman, Judith L. 1992. *Trauma and Recovery*. New York: Basic Books.

Herman, Judith L., J. C. Perry, and B. A. van der Kolk. 1989. "Childhood Trauma in Borderline Personality Disorder." *American Journal of Psychiatry* 146 (4): 460–465.

Hicks, D. Emily. 1991. *Border Writing : The Multidimensional Text*. Minneapolis: University of Minnesota Press.

Hoch, Paul, and Phillip Polatin. 1949. "Pseudoneurotic Forms of Schizophrenia." *Psychiatric Quarterly* 23: 248–276.

Hoffman, Irwin. 1991. "Discussion: Toward a Social Constructivist View of the Psychoanalytic Situation." *Psychoanalytic Dialogues* 1: 74–105.

hooks, bell. 1991. Interview in *Angry Women*. Eds. A. Juno and V. Vale. San Francisco: Re/search Publications.

Hyler, Steven E., and Bella Schanzer. 1997. "Using Commercially Available Films to Teach About Borderline Personality Disorder." *Bulletin of the Menninger Clinic* 61 (4): 458–468.

Ingleby, David. 1985. "Professionals as Socializers: The 'Psy Complex.'" *Research in Law, Deviance and Social Control* 7: 79–109.

Irigaray, Luce. 1985. *The Speculum of the Other Woman*. Trans. G. C. Gill. Ithaca, N.Y.: Cornell University Press.

Jimenez, Mary Ann. 1997. "Gender and Psychiatry: Psychiatric Conceptions of Mental Disorders in Women, 1960–1994." *Affilia* 12 (2): 154–175.

Juno, Andrea, and V. Vale, eds. 1991. *Angry Women*. San Francisco: Re/search Publications.

Kahane, Claire. 1985. "Introduction: Part Two." In *In Dora's Case: Freud-Hysteria-Feminism*. Ed. C. Bernheimer and C. Kahane. New York: Columbia University Press.

Kaplan, Marcie. 1983. "A Woman's View of the DSM-III." *American Psychologist* 38 (7): 786–792.

Kaysen, Susan. 1993. *Girl, Interrupted*. New York: Turtle Bay Books.

Kohut, Heinz. 1977. *The Restoration of the Self*. New York: International Universities Press.

Kornreich, Jennifer. 1997. "Borderlines." *Long Island Voice* 1 (24): 14–17.

Kovel, Joel. 1988. "A Critique of DSM-III." *Research in Law, Deviance, and Social Control* 9: 127–146.

Kristeva, Julia. 1995. *New Maladies of the Soul*. New York: Columbia University Press.

Lakoff, George. 1987. *Women, Fire, and Dangerous Things: What Categories Reveal About the Mind*. Chicago: University of Chicago Press.

Lazar, Norman D. 1973. "Nature and Significance of Changes in Patients in a Psychoanalytic Clinic." *Psychoanalytic Quarterly* 42 (4): 579–600.

Lazare, Aaron. 1971. "The Hysterical Character in Psychoanalytic Theory." *Archives of General Psychiatry* 25: 131–137.

Leichtman, Martin. 1989. "Evolving Concepts of Borderline Personality Disorders." *Bulletin of the Menninger Clinic* 53 (3): 229–249.

Lerner, Harriet. 1988. "Special Issues for Women in Psychotherapy." In *Women in Therapy*, by H. Lerner. Northvale, N.J.: Jason Aronson.

Lesser, Ronnie C. 1996. "'All That's Solid Melts Into Air': Deconstructing Some Psychoanalytic Facts." *Contemporary Psychoanalysis* 32 (1): 5–23.

Lévi-Strauss, Claude. 1969. *The Elementary Structures of Kinship*. Trans. James Harle Bell, John Richard von Sturmer, and Rodney Needham. Boston: Beacon Press.

Linehan, Marcia. 1993. *Cognitive-Behavioral Treatment of Borderline Personality Disorder*. New York: Guilford Press.

Lunbeck, Elizabeth. 1994. *The Psychiatric Persuasion: Knowledge, Gender and Power in Modern America*. Princeton, N.J.: Princeton University Press.

Mack, John E. 1975. "Borderline States: An Historical Perspective." In *Borderline States in Psychiatry: An Historical Perspective*. Ed. J. E. Mack. New York: Grune and Stratton.

McNamee, Sheila, and Kenneth J. Gergen, eds. 1992. *Therapy as Social Construction*. Thousand Oaks, Calif.: Sage.

Maines, David R. 1993. "Narrative's Moment and Sociology's Phenomena: Toward a Narrative Sociology." *Sociological Quarterly* 34 (1): 17–38.

Malcolm, Janet. 1982. *Psychoanalysis: The Impossible Profession*. New York: Alfred A. Knopf.

Marcus, Stephen. 1985. "Freud and Dora: Story, History, Case History." In *In Dora's Case: Freud-Hysteria-Feminism*. Eds. C. Bernheimer and C. Kahane. New York: Columbia University Press.

Meissner, William W. 1984. *The Borderline Spectrum: Differential Diagnosis and Development Issues*. New York: Jason Aronson.

Millon, Theodore. 1983. "The DSM III: An Insider's Perspective." *American Psychologist* 38: 804–814.

———.1987. "On the Genesis and Prevalence of the Borderline Personality Disorder: A Social Learning Thesis." *Journal of Personality Disorders* 1 (4): 354–372.

Mitchell, Juliet, and Jacqueline Rose. 1982. *Feminine Sexuality: Jacques Lacan and the École Freudienne*. New York: W. W. Norton.

Mitchell, Stephen A. 1988. *Relational Concepts in Psychoanalysis: An Integration*. Cambridge, Mass.: Harvard University Press.

Moi, Toril. 1985. "Representation of Patriarchy: Sexuality and Epistemology in Freud's Dora." In *In Dora's Case: Freud-Hysteria-Feminism*. Eds. C. Bernheimer and C. Kahane. New York: Columbia University Press.

Nadelson, Theodore. 1977. "Borderline Rage and the Therapist's Response." *American Journal of Psychiatry* 134 (7): 748–751.

O'Hanlon, William Hudson. 1992. "History Becomes Her Story: Collaborative Solution-Oriented Therapy of the After-Effects of Sexual Abuse." In *Therapy as Social Construction*. Eds. S. McNamee and K. J. Gergen. Thousand Oaks, Calif.: Sage.

Ong, Aiwa. 1988. "The Production of Possession: Spirits and the Multinational Corporation in Malaysia." *American Ethnologist* 15: 28–42.

Paris, Joel. 1991. "Personality Disorders, Parasuicide, and Culture." *Transcultural Psychiatric Research Review* 28 (1): 25–39.

Perry, J. Christopher, and Gerald L. Klerman. 1978. "The Borderline Patient: A Comparative Analysis of Four Sets of Diagnostic Criteria." *Archives of General Psychiatry* 35: 141–150.

Peters, Larry G. 1994. "Rites of Passage and the Borderline Syndrome: Perspectives in Transpersonal Anthropology." *Anthropology of Consciousness* 5 (1): 1–15.

Plath, Sylvia. 1971. *The Bell Jar*. New York: Harper and Row.

Polkinghorne, Donald E. 1988. *Narrative Knowing in the Human Sciences*. Albany: State University of New York Press.

Ramas, Maria. 1985. "Freud's Dora: Dora's Hysteria." In *In Dora's Case: Freud-Hysteria-Feminism*. Eds. C. Bernheimer and C. Kahane. New York: Columbia University Press.

Rangell, Leo. 1955. "Scientific Proceedings: Panel Reports. The Borderline Case." *Journal of the American Psychoanalytic Association* 3: 285–298.

Reiser, David E., and Hanna Levenson. 1984. "Abuses of the Borderline Diagnosis: A Clinical Problem with Teaching Opportunities." *American Journal of Psychiatry* 141 (12): 1528–1532.

Reissman, Catherine. 1990. *Divorce Talk: Women and Men Make Sense of Personal Relationships.* New Brunswick, N.J.: Rutgers University Press.

Rich, Charles. 1978. "Borderline Diagnoses." *American Journal of Psychiatry* 135 (11): 1399–1401.

Richardson, Laurel. 1995. "Narrative and Sociology." In *Representation in Ethnography.* Ed. J. Van Maanen. Thousand Oaks, Calif.: Sage.

Riviere, J. 1929. "Womanliness as Masquerade." *International Journal of Psychoanalysis* 10: 303–313.

Romanyshyn, Robert. 1989. *Technology as Dream and Symptom.* New York: Routledge.

Rose, Nikolas. 1996. *Inventing Ourselves: Psychology, Power and Personhood.* Cambridge, Mass.: Cambridge University Press.

Ross, Manuel. 1976. "The Borderline Diathesis." *International Review of Psycho-Analysis* 3: 305–321.

Rosse, Irving. 1886. "Clinical Evidences of Borderland Insanity." In *Essential Papers on Borderline Disorders: One Hundred Years at the Border.* Ed. M. H. Stone. New York: New York University Press.

Rubin, Gayle. 1975. "The Traffic in Women: Notes on the Political Economy of Sex." In *Toward an Anthropology of Women.* Ed. R. R. Reiter. New York: Monthly Review Press.

Ryan, Michael. 1982. *Marxism and Deconstruction: A Critical Articulation.* Baltimore: Johns Hopkins University Press.

Samuels, Andrew. 1988. "Gender and the Borderline." In *The Borderline Personality in Analysis.* Ed. N. Schwartz-Salant and M. Stein. Wilmette, Ill.: Chiron.

Sass, Louis A. 1982. "The Borderline Personality." *New York Times Magazine,* 22 August, 12–66.

———.1988. "The Self and Its Vicissitudes: An 'Archaeological' Study of the Psychoanalytic Avant-Garde." *Social Research* 55 (4): 551–607.

———.1994. "The Epic of Disbelief: The Postmodernist Turn in Psychoanalysis." *Partisan Review* 61 (1): 96–110.

Satow, Roberta. 1980. "Where Has All the Hysteria Gone?" *Psychoanalytic Review* 66: 463–478.

Schafer, Roy. 1989. "Narratives of the Self." In *Psychoanalysis: Toward the Second Century.* Eds. A. M. Cooper, O. F. Kernberg, and E. S. Person. New Haven, Conn.: Yale University Press.

Schwartz-Salant, Nathan. 1987. "The Dead Self in Borderline Personality Disorders." In *Pathologies of the Modern Self: Postmodern Studies on Narcissism, Schizophrenia, and Depression.* Ed. D. M. Levin. New York: New York University Press.

———.1989. *Borderline Personality: Vision and Healing.* Wilmette, Ill.: Chiron.

Showalter, Elaine. 1985. *The Female Malady: Women, Madness, and English Culture 1830–1980.* New York: Penguin.

———.1990. *Sexual Anarchy: Gender and Culture at the Fin de Siècle.* New York: Viking.

Singer, Melvin. 1977a. "The Experience of Emptiness in Narcissistic and Borderline States I: The Struggle for a Sense of Self and the Potential for Suicide." *International Review of Psycho-Analysis* 4: 459–469.

———.1977b. "The Experience of Emptiness in Narcissistic and Borderline States: II. The Struggle for a Sense of Self and the Potential for Suicide." In *International Review of Psycho-Analysis* 4: 471–479.

Smith, Dorothy. 1990. *Texts, Facts and Femininity: Exploring the Relations of Ruling.* New York: Routledge.

Smith-Rosenberg, Carroll. 1972. "The Hysterical Woman: Sex Roles and Role Conflict in 19th-Century America." *Social Research* 39: 652–678.

Spence, Donald P. 1984. *Narrative Truth and Historical Truth: Meaning and Interpretation in Psychoanalysis.* New York: W. W. Norton.

Spitzer, Robert L., Janet B. W. Williams, and Andrew Skodol. 1980. "DSM-III: The Major Achievements and an Overview." *American Journal of Psychiatry* 137 (2): 151–164.

Sprock, J., R. Blashfield, and B. Smith. 1990. "Gender Weighting of DSM-III-R Personality Disorder Criteria." *American Journal of Psychiatry* 147: 586–590.

Stein, Martin. 1989. "The Treatment of a Low Level Borderline Personality Disorder." *Issues in Ego Psychology* 13 (2): 124–139.

Stern, Adolph. 1938. "Psychoanalytic Investigation of and Therapy in the Border Line Group of Neuroses." *Psychoanalytic Quarterly* 7: 467–489.

Stone, Michael H., ed. 1986. *Essential Papers on Borderline Disorders: One Hundred Years at the Border.* New York: New York University Press.

Strong, Marilee. 1998. *A Bright Red Scream: Self-Mutilation and the Language of Pain.* New York: Viking.

Susko, Michael A. 1994. "Caseness and Narrative: Contrasting Approaches to People Who are Psychiatrically Labeled." *Journal of Mind and Behavior.* 15 (1–2): 87–112.

Swartz, Marvin, Dan Blazer, Linda George, and Idee Winfield. 1990. "Estimating the Prevalence of Borderline Personality Disorder in the Community." *Journal of Personality Disorders* 4 (3): 257–272.

Theweleit, Klaus. 1987. *Male Fantasies: Volume I: Women, Floods, Bodies, History.* Trans. S. Conway. Minneapolis: University of Minnesota Press.

Trull, Timothy J., Thomas Widiger, and Pamela Guthrie. 1990. "Categorical Versus Dimensional Status of Borderline Personality Disorder." *Journal of Abnormal Psychology* 99 (1): 40–48.

Turner, Bryan. 1987. *Medical Power and Social Knowledge.* London: Sage.

Ussher, Jane. 1992. *Women's Madness: Misogyny or Mental Illness?* Amherst: University of Massachusetts Press.

Waldinger, Robert J., and John G. Gunderson. 1987. *Effective Psychotherapy with Borderline Patients: Case Studies.* New York: Macmillan.

Wanklin, Jane. 1997. *Let Me Make It Good: A Chronicle of My Life with Borderline Personality Disorder.* Oakville, Ontario, Canada: Mosaic Press.

Warren, Carol A. B. 1987. *Madwives: Schizophrenic Women in the 1950s.* New Brunswick, N.J.: Rutgers University Press.

Wedding, Danny, and Mary Ann Boyd. 1999. *Movies and Mental Illness: Using Films to Understand Psychopathology.* New York: McGraw-Hill.

White, Michael, and David Epston. 1990. *Narrative Means to Therapeutic Ends.* New York: W. W. Norton.

Yalom, Irvin D. 1989. "Therapeutic Monogamy." In *Love's Executioner and Other Tales of Psychotherapy.* New York: Basic Books.

Yalom, Irvin D., and Ginny Elkin. 1974. *Every Day Gets a Little Closer: A Twice-Told Therapy.* New York: Basic Books.

Zilboorg, Gregory. 1941. "Ambulatory Schizophrenias." *Psychiatry* 4: 149–155.

Index

Abend, Sander M., 95, 111–113

abject: autobiographical reflection on, 151; clients as, 86–87; concept of, 85–86, 101; masquerade vs., 122–123. *See also* masks/masking

abnormality, use of term, 47

addiction, 56

adolescence, 149, 153, 155, 164. *See also Girl, Interrupted* (Kaysen); *Let Me Make It Good* (Wanklin)

African Americans, emotions of, 76

age, as factor, 13

aggression: as BPD symptom, 8, 89, 96–97, 115; fantasy linked to, 107. *See also* self-mutilation; suicidal acts

alcohol abuse, 56, 156–157

Alexander, Franz, 48

American Psychiatric Association, 49, 57

Anafranil, 156

anger. *See* rage

anorexia-bulimia: control in, 154, 164; as embodiment of body/mind split, 153–154; as expression of self-hatred and depression, 151; self-mutilation associated with, 158–159; as sign of societal dysfunction, 29–30, 200; sources of, 135–136, 158, 162, 163

antisocial personality disorder, 62, 71, 74–75

anxiety: narcissism as source of, 50; in pan-neurosis, 65; to relieve

emptiness, 100, 105–106

appearance: as masking, 124–128; as off-center, 92–93, 116; racial codings of, 123

Aronson, Thomas A., 39, 41–42, 55

artificiality, as theme, 121–123, 130–131

"as if" personality, 64–65, 122

assassinations, 152, 164

assemblage, concept of, 15

asylum, emerging need for, 45. *See also* hospitalization

autobiography: abject in, 151; function of, 144–145; of lost self, 128–133; power issues and, 201; reconstructing trauma in, 161–167; on subject/object dichotomy, 119–120. *See also Girl, Interrupted* (Kaysen); *Let Me Make It Good* (Wanklin)

autonomous self: borderline double and, 139–140; effacement of, 131–132; madness of, 172; repression of, 133–134, 136–137

Babener, Liana, 171

Basic Instinct (film), 170

Bauer, Ida (Dora case), 23–25, 90, 179–181, 182

Beauvoir, Simone de, 84

Becker, Dana: on borderline symptoms, 27; on borderline terminology, 38, 62, 202, 203; on feminization of borderline, 4, 5, 8–9, 69–72, 78; on

social conditions: as causative agent, 163; literalization of, 28; as narrative's context, 22–25; symptoms as response to, 27–30, 152–153, 164–165. *See also* culture; gender relations and roles

Social Darwinism, 46–47

social deviance: insanity linked to, 45–48, 56; transgressing boundaries as, 123–124. *See also* marginalization; promiscuity; resistance; self-mutilation; theft

socialization, of women, 205–208

social self, 135

social violence, 29–30

society: alienation from, 147; assassinations in, 152–153; dysfunction of, 29–30; identity problems in context of, 10, 12–13; instability of, 12–13, 82; narrative's role in, 17; as stress source, 151–152; woman's position in, 79–80, 81–87, 158. *See also* culture; gender relations and roles; norms

sociopaths, men diagnosed as, 74, 77

soldiers, fluid metaphors and, 102–103

somatization disorder, 67, 73

spirit possession, 27–28

splitting: of borderline double, 138–143, 165–166; description of, 54; origins of, 128; rage/resistance and, 190–191; trauma and, 68, 160–161. *See also* dissociative states; fragmentation

Stein, Martin: masks of femininity and, 122–128, 165; on off-center appearance, 92–93, 116

Stern, Adolph: BPD case described by, 49–50; on neurosis/psychosis border, 3, 32, 38, 48

stigma, of insanity, 150

Stone, Michael, 5, 52–54, 64

storytelling. *See* autobiography; case narratives; narrative

stress, societal sources of, 151–152

Strong, Marilee, 156, 158–159, 161, 163

Studies in Hysteria (Freud and Breuer), 18

subject, gendering of, 81–87

subjectification, 15, 28

subjectivities: complexity of, 165–167; context of constructing, 163–165; crisis in, 9–12; excising part of, 147–148; feminine embodiment disavowed in, 134; masculine as model of, 83–85; as multiple/relational, 209–211. *See also* gender relations and roles

subject/object dichotomy: female division in, 119–120; woman's standpoint in, 82–87, 116. *See also* body/mind split

suicidal acts: autobiographical reflections on, 144; borderline double and, 141; desolation as precursor to, 147–148; pregnancy equated with, 145; as symptom, 64; treatment for, 135, 157, 177–178. *See also* para-suicide

superficiality, as theme, 121–123

surveyor/surveyed, 119, 158

Susko, Michael, 144–145

symptoms: aggression as, 8, 89, 96–97, 115; clinical case studies as formal interpretation of, 17–18; contradictions in, 177; as defenses, 103; description of general, 30–31, 50, 54–55, 128–129, 138, 151, 170; feminist analysis of, 200–202; misogynist view of, 171–172; multiplicity of, 33, 39–40; mutability of, 70, 129; official list of, 61; para-suicide as, 13, 14; primary, 70, 98, 172; as response to social conditions, 27–30; search for origins of, 152; as self-healing attempts, 14, 156, 161; social construction of, 197; text as/as text, 7, 22–25, 26–31; theft as, 179. *See also* empty self; fragmentation; marginalization; rage; self-mutilation; unstable self

Taubin, Amy, 172

About the Author

Janet Wirth-Cauchon is an associate professor of sociology at Drake University. In addition to gender and mental illness, her research and teaching interests include feminist theory, identity and culture, and the body and technology.